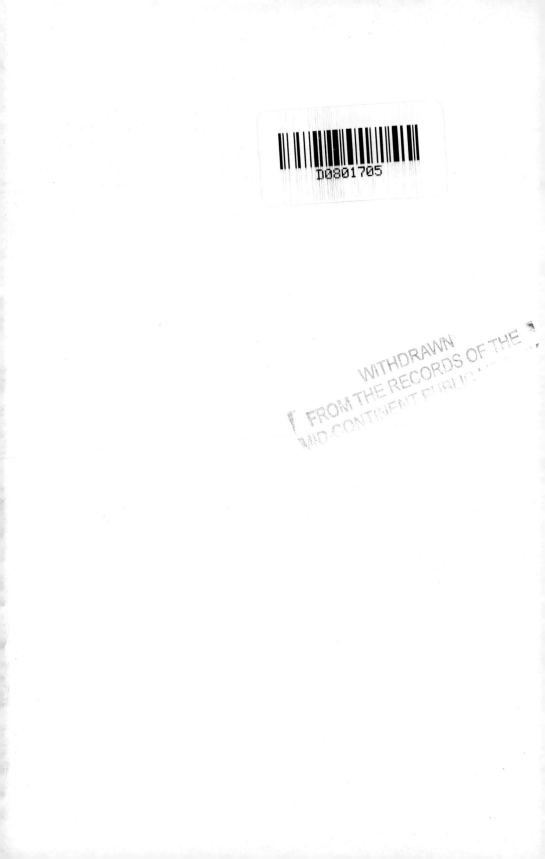

MOM IN THE MIRROR

Mom in the Mirror

*Body Image, Beauty,
and Life after Pregnancy*

DENA CABRERA
AND
EMILY T. WIERENGA

ROWMAN & LITTLEFIELD PUBLISHERS, INC.
Lanham • Boulder • New York • Toronto • Plymouth, UK

Published by Rowman & Littlefield Publishers, Inc.
A wholly owned subsidary of The Rowman & Littlefield Publishing Group, Inc.
4501 Forbes Boulevard, Suite 200, Lanham, Maryland 20706
www.rowman.com

10 Thornbury Road, Plymouth PL6 7PP, United Kingdom

Distributed by National Book Network

Copyright © 2013 by Dena Cabrera and Emily T. Wierenga

British Library Cataloguing in Publication Information Available

Library of Congress Cataloging-in-Publication Data

Cabrera, Dena, 1969–
  Mom in the mirror : body image, beauty, and life after pregnancy / Dena
Cabrera and Emily T. Wierenga.
    p. cm
  Includes bibliographical references and index.
  ISBN 978-1-4422-1865-9 (hbk. : alk. paper) — ISBN 978-1-4422-1867-3
(electronic) (print) 1. Body image. 2. Beauty, Personal. 3. Self-esteem. 4.
Pregnancy—Psychological aspects. 5. Motherhood—Psychological aspects. I.
Wierenga, Emily T., 1980– II. Title.
  BF697.5.B63C33 2013
  155.3'33—dc23
                                                          2012039576

Printed in the United States of America

This book is dedicated to our mothers. We love you.

mother

soft hands flowered apron you
stand in doorway sunlight spilling 'round
you
mother

soft music gentle prayers you
love to laugh hate to stare proper british
woman
mother

soft heart big worries you
try to release not letting go begging stay! yet i leave
you
mother

soft tears washing face your
big blue eyes full of grace i love you need you try to be
you
mother

—*e. wierenga*

Giving birth produces life in more than one sense. It's the baby powder, milky-breathed spirit found in the softest limbs you've ever felt, and it's the respect a man feels for his wife as he watches her give up her body for another. And it's the deep-rooted, soul-satisfying feeling of knowing you were born for more than the mirror. That you were born to see the face of God in your child, and to know that you yourself are a miracle.

CONTENTS

Foreword by Emme   ix

Introduction   xi

1   Our Bodies, Ourselves: The Dissatisfied Generation   1

2   A Bruised Beginning: From Girlhood to Adolescence   17

3   From Bruised to Broken: When Adolescent Turns Adult   27

4   Before and After: The Effects of Pregnancy   35

5   Change, Acceptance, and More Change:
    Embracing Motherhood   49

6   The Sleepless Wife: How to Balance Marriage
    and Motherhood   63

7   Beyond Breast Milk (or Formula): The Challenges of
    Feeding Children   73

8   Food from Heaven: Spiritual Nourishment for You
    and Your Family   89

9   Like Mother, Like Daughter: Your Personal Legacy   105

10 Being the Mirror: How to Inspire Beauty in
    Our Children   117

CONTENTS

11 The Anxious Mother: Using Food, Exercise, or Work
as an Escape   135

12 Friendly Competition: Your Relationship with
Other Women   151

13 As They Grow: Your Changing Role as a Mom and
a Woman   161

14 Getting Help: Hope and a Cure   173

15 Identity Crisis: Discovering True Self-Worth   187

Acknowledgments   197

Appendix   199

Notes   207

Selected Bibliography   217

Index   219

About the Authors   227

FOREWORD

I am often asked to review books relating to body image, self-esteem, and eating disorders, but when Dr. Dena Cabrera and I first spoke about *Mom in the Mirror*, I knew something groundbreaking was about to be birthed.

Rarely has the topic of a mother's body image been successfully addressed or delved into. Sadly, the concept of self-love is hardly spoken of at all.

Mom in the Mirror pulls back the covers to combine practical lessons by Dr. Cabrera with honest insights by coauthor Emily Wierenga, a recovered anorexic and mother of four boys, creating, as the book describes it, "a unique self-help narrative that will inspire mothers to turn inward for their value and worth."

Be done with denying food, pretending to feel full, convincing yourself you don't need help, or telling those you love that everything's okay, when clearly everything is not. No more playing with your mind, stretching the truth, or hiding yourself. You deserve a lot more of what this life has to offer, as do the children who look to you for guidance at every turn.

Break the chains of self-loathing, unrealistic expectations, social pressures, familial perceptions of beauty, and body bashing, and be free in the here and now. Learn to love, starting with yourself.

We live in a society that demonizes fat; meanwhile, we are more overweight than ever before. Every day at least ten million women deny themselves acceptance and love by abusing food in some way, shape, or form. Clearly, something is wrong.

What if we dug in and reconnected with our mind, body, and spirit as mothers? Don't you think it's time to reclaim the life that is undeniably ours to live? A life that isn't made in the image of some ad campaign or movie, selling us a shortchanged bill of goods? A life that isn't discussed and arranged on corporate America's conference-room tables?

I know you've been waiting for a book like this to help alleviate your pain, explain the insanity you've been living, and to be your friend, your confidant, and support. Welcome to the answers you've been looking for, some good hard facts to lead you to your personal worth, and the power to change.

Your children will never be able to thank you enough, let alone their children, and so forth. It all starts with you. Allow yourself to begin life anew, starting now.

Emme (Melissa Aronson)
Author, Television Host, and Plus-Size Supermodel
EmmeNation.com

INTRODUCTION

Nothing changes a person like giving birth. Just ask any of the 85.4 million mothers in the United States.[1] This turning inside out so that another person might live excavates and transforms and inspires. But before we become mothers (and even afterward), we're women first.

There are women who don't like their reflection in the mirror because for some reason, the crow's-feet and widow's peak and thin lips say something about their value and their worth. Looks have become synonymous with identity. As a result, a nation of women with body image issues is struggling to inspire a generation of daughters.

Seventy-five percent of females aged twenty-five to forty-five exhibit disordered eating behaviors. Three out of four women have an unhealthy relationship with food or their bodies (including the 10 percent who meet criteria for diagnosable eating disorders such as anorexia, bulimia, and binge eating disorder).

And there's more:

- 67 percent of women (excluding those with actual eating disorders) are trying to lose weight
- 53 percent of dieters are already at a healthy weight and still trying to lose weight
- 39 percent of women say concerns about what they eat or weigh interfere with their happiness
- 37 percent regularly skip meals to try to lose weight
- 27 percent would be "extremely upset" if they gained just five pounds

- 26 percent cut out entire food groups
- 16 percent have dieted on 1,000 calories a day or less
- 13 percent smoke to lose weight
- 12 percent eat regularly when they're not hungry, and 49 percent sometimes do[2]

Because most women spend their lives attempting to change their bodies, it's not surprising that adding postpregnancy pounds and the challenges of parenting only exacerbate issues with weight, body image, and disordered eating. We're not just talking about women with "clinical" eating disorders. Every day, tens of millions of women deny their bodies the food they need—regardless of whether they're trying to lose five pounds or fifty. And no matter how hard we try to inspire health, wholeness, and confidence in our children, unless we love ourselves, they won't love themselves, either.

MOM IN THE MIRROR

So how do we deal with the challenges of parenting, in addition to our own unrealistic expectations, media influences, perceived pressures from those around us, and a culture that demonizes fat (even though more Americans are overweight than ever before)? *Mom in the Mirror* is a biological, psychological, social, cultural, and spiritual response to this question. Within its pages, Dr. Dena Cabrera, former staff psychologist at Remuda Ranch and currently the executive clinical director of training and education at the Rosewood Institute, combines her expertise with the personal experience of Emily T. Wierenga, a recovered anorexic and mother of four boys, to create a unique self-help narrative that will inspire mothers to turn inward for their value and worth. *Mom in the Mirror* provides insight, support, and the information necessary to help readers overcome damaging lifestyle habits and self-esteem struggles. Readers will learn how to improve the way they eat, live, feel, and parent, thereby increasing their happiness, confidence, and self-esteem both as mothers *and* women.

There are countless resources aimed at promoting health in one's children and guiding parents with eating-disordered offspring. There are also plenty of diet books to help new mothers lose postpregnancy weight. But *Mom in the Mirror* is different; its purpose is twofold. It aims to help women separate the truth from the lies about who they are, and to subsequently improve relationships with their bodies, their families, and their Creator.

THE AUTHORS

Having battled anorexia nervosa both as a child and as an adult, Emily was told by doctors that due to the damage she'd done to her body, she probably wouldn't be able to conceive. Today, Emily and her husband, Trenton, are the parents of four boys, two of them biological. An artist, musician, and freelance journalist, Emily credits the miracle of giving birth with saving her perception of herself, her marriage, and her faith.

Becoming a parent also affected Dena through her work as a therapist and an eating disorder specialist. When her daughter, Alexis, was still an infant, Dena was counseling a patient who had battled anorexia for five years. Gloria was the mother of three boys, ages seven, nine, and eleven; she told Dena that parenting was a complete joy for her. She cherished every minute with her darling sons, who were perfect in every way. Dena, meanwhile, was exhausted, sleep deprived, and insecure about her role and abilities as a new parent. She remembers thinking, "How in the world are you parenting your children while battling an eating disorder?" Dena was struggling with just one child—and she wasn't dealing with a potentially fatal condition.

Eventually it became clear that Gloria was in denial, not only about her illness, but about her feelings toward parenting in general. When she finally admitted to Dena that she was struggling as a mom, a role complicated by anorexia, Dena realized that body image was an issue *all* women struggled with—mothers included. You don't have to have a diagnosable eating disorder to need this book. Millions of mothers wrestle daily, not only with portion size or nutritious meal plans, but with a negative response to their reflection in the mirror. If that's you, we want to help. With God as our guide, we will improve how you feel about your body, how you approach food, how you parent, and ultimately, how you live.

So let's get started.

OUR BODIES, OURSELVES

The Dissatisfied Generation

You can take no credit for beauty at sixteen. But if you are beautiful at sixty, it will be your soul's own doing.

—Marie Stopes

WHAT IT MEANS TO BE A WOMAN

This business of being a woman in the twenty-first century—of balancing motherhood, marriage, and career with an airbrushed smile—is hard. The anxiety of it all makes us wallow in a carton of ice cream. "To be a woman is to have a body image problem," writes Mary Pipher, PhD.[1] As females, we are born people pleasers who, along with giving birth to children, give birth to enormous bouts of self-doubt. We take pride in this "mother guilt" that keeps us up all hours of the night and tears at the fabric of our marriages. It makes us jealous of each other, unable to connect with our children, fearful of the future, and paranoid of rejection. To deal with our tormented souls, we find comfort in fast food and Twinkies, or we starve ourselves in an attempt to feel like we're in control. We spend hours on the treadmill, chasing our guilt. But guilt always runs faster, and ultimately, it leaves us spent and exhausted. "Most women will do anything, including becoming mental patients, to help their families," says Pipher.[2]

So we bear the brunt of the world in an attempt to save it, but this is not, in fact, doing anyone any good because we cannot save the world. And we cannot save ourselves. We can only learn to love. We learn to love by dying to ourselves. By dying to what we thought we were worth (nothing) and accepting what we *are* worth (everything). By rejecting the world's mantra that we are what we look like, and believing, instead, that we are lovely simply because we exist. Yet it's easier to believe the negative, and so we pinch our stomachs in disgust, spend hours at the gym, put other women down, and throw up our dinner.

"It's not very easy to grow up into a woman," says C. JoyBell C., author of *The Sun Is Snowing: Poetry and Prose by C. JoyBell C.* "We are always taught, almost bombarded, with ideals of what we should be at every age in our lives . . . I want to be able to say that there are four things admirable for a woman to be, at any age! Whether you are four or 45 or 19! It's always wonderful to be elegant, it's always fashionable to have grace, it's always glamorous to be brave, and it's always important to own a delectable perfume! Yes, wearing a beautiful fragrance is in style at any age!"[3]

It's also admirable, sometimes, to put ourselves first. Because how can we serve our families—how can we love our husbands, our children—if we don't love ourselves first? And how many of us can say we love ourselves? Most of us can admit to loving *things about* ourselves, but do we love our *selves*? The parts that make us *us*?

"A woman's happiness is in throwing everything away to live for love," says Ai Yazawa in *Paradise Kiss, Volume 5*.[4] But this living for love does not mean throwing away our dreams and desires. No, it means fully entering ourselves, while ridding ourselves of any preconceived notions about beauty and value and worth. It means embracing our crooked noses, our snorting laughter, the stretch marks, saggy boobs, tea-bag eyes, and warty feet. It means accepting our humanness, but it also means more than that. It means approaching ourselves like author Anne Lamott does: with kindness and laughter. "Age has given me what I was looking for my entire life," Lamott writes. "It has given me *me*. It has provided time and experience and failures and triumphs and time-tested friends who have helped me step into the shape that was waiting for me. I fit into me now."⁵

We each have a shape. It may not be perfect, but it's *ours*; it is a unique space in history to fill. But it's up to us to take care of this shape, to respect and honor the role we've been given.

Blogger Brandee Shafer has been heavyset her entire adult life, her weight ranging anywhere from 150 to 205 pounds; her pant size, from 11 to 16. Until recently, she was perfectly comfortable in her own skin. "I'm known for saying (and meaning) things like: 'Those Peanut Butter M&M's were totally worth it!'" she writes. "And—if I'm to be *completely* honest with you—my extra weight has made me feel mostly sturdy . . . like a Morgan mare I used to ride."

However, during her pregnancy with her daughter, Brandee was diagnosed with gestational diabetes. "The nausea was bad," she writes. "The dizziness was worse. For months, I cooked and washed dishes while sitting on a stool. [One day] I passed out in a Dollar Tree." In addition to tiring easily, Brandee experienced dramatic sugar highs and lows: "I used to smoke, and my cravings for sugar are at least as intense as my cravings for nicotine used to be."

And then she had a miscarriage. "Now, don't misunderstand," explains Brandee. "I've no reason to believe my miscarriage had anything to do with my weight or my eating habits; however, for the first time, I realized my body's capability for failure."⁶

It is this capability for failure that so many of us women struggle with. We lose ourselves in depression, food, weigh scales, and dieting because we don't want to face our brokenness. And the older we get, and the more children (and stretch marks) we acquire, the more broken we become. Hence, the more we try to lose ourselves.

"On my forty-ninth birthday, I decided that all of life was hopeless, and I would eat myself to death," writes Lamott. Then, she adds, "These are desert days . . . [but] Father Tom loves the desert. A number of my friends do. They love the skies that pull you into infinity, like the ocean. They love the silence, and how, if you listen long enough, the pulse of the desert begins to sound like the noise your finger makes when you run it around the rim of a crystal glass. They love the scary beauty—snakes, lizards, scorpions, the kestrels and hawks. They love the mosaics of water-washed pebbles on the desert floor, small rocks that cast huge shadows, a shoot of vegetation here, a wildflower there."[7]

This book is about learning, as women, to love the desert days—the broken and the hard places, the scary beauty within us. It's about finding the wildflowers in our soul and fertilizing them and allowing them to seed, and to erupt, full into joy.

A LOT OF UNHAPPY, HUNGRY WOMEN

What do you see when you look in the mirror? Do you see a mother? A wife? A woman? Or do you see, to put it kindly, a "mess"? Do you see saggy breasts, lumpy thighs, a flabby stomach, hips you hate? Is this a body you are constantly at war with? Are you at a weight that falls far short of your own ideal, much less society's?

As Westernized women, we are obsessed with our bodies, and with changing them. Studies show that 89 percent of women want to lose weight, while 60 percent are on a diet at any given time.[8] That's a lot of unhappy, hungry women. Women in general deal with myriad eating and body image issues. But as a psychologist who specializes in helping women with eating disorders, Dena knows firsthand that moms have it particularly tough. After all, they're experiencing a tremendous amount of responsibility and pressure, having undergone an enormous transformation from woman-sans-child to mother. No matter what anyone tells you, you're never quite prepared for the change that such a small person can cause.

The poet William Ross Wallace famously wrote, "The hand that rocks the cradle rules the world." Unfortunately, the majority of moms feel anything but powerful, and they have an ever-present, oppressive item on their lengthy to-do list: "lose weight."

Michelle, forty-two, admits that dieting and exercising have ruled her life. She told Dena that she is still "trying to lose the baby weight." When Dena asked Michelle how old her baby was, she replied, "Thirteen." It wasn't a joke. Michelle gets up every morning, pinching her stomach and feeling disgusted with herself. She always wants to be thinner and is constantly dieting. But if you saw her, you'd never know it. She's slim and close to underweight.

Like Michelle, many mothers suffer in silence. Others join up with their friends to cheer each other on to attain their perfect weights, whether that means losing ten pounds or fifty. On the surface, it seems harmless—but is it?

DIETING VERSUS DISORDERED EATING

The survey mentioned in the introduction, conducted in 2008 by the University of North Carolina in collaboration with *Self* magazine, found that three-quarters of the female population eats unhealthily. These findings were not limited to one group: unhealthy eating behaviors were identified in diverse ethnic backgrounds including Hispanic, Caucasian, African American/black, and Asian women. It was shocking to learn that 60 percent of women (excluding those with diagnosed eating disorders) are trying to lose weight, while 53 percent of those dieters are already at a healthy body mass index. We find that statistic both sad and scary—but at the same time, it doesn't surprise us. Dena has been treating women with eating disorders for over sixteen years, and has learned the problem goes far beyond women with diagnosable eating disorders.

Have you ever skipped a meal to save calories, or purposely ignored your hunger signals? Have you ever forced yourself to exercise, not for the physical pleasure of moving your body, but to burn off a few hundred calories? Have you found yourself grabbing the sagging flesh around your stomach in despair, wishing you could just cut it off or afford a tummy tuck? Or perhaps you've admitted, "I hate my thighs," or "My stomach is disgusting," or "I am so fat"?

And have your children heard you?

DISCONNECTED AND DISGUSTED

Linda, thirty-six, is a mother of three boys under the age of ten. Because of her obsession with dieting, Linda does not eat meals with her family. She can't even remember the last time she sat and ate with her children; she only eats alone, at night. She says that, as a mother, "I am just going through the motions. I feel so disconnected." Her relationship with food and with her body is linked to her disconnectedness with her children and husband—the people she loves the most. Yet she doesn't know how to change. Meanwhile, she's losing time she'll never get back. Soon her kids will grow up and leave home.

Focusing on weight, shape, and food can take over your life and imprison you. We're not just talking about the time and energy you spend worrying about what you're going to eat (or not eat) at your next meal, or beating yourself up for "blowing it" when you slip off the diet. We're talking about *not being present in your day-to-day life*, both as a woman and as a mom.

Remember the tear-jerking scene in *E.T.* when E.T. is saying good-bye to Elliott before going home? E.T. expresses his pain at having to leave Elliott by tapping his chest, motioning toward Elliott, and saying, "Ouch." Elliott repeats the movement and the word. Even after seeing the movie six times, Dena always cries during this scene. This is a good analogy regarding our connection with our children. We hurt when they hurt; we feel it deeply in our bodies and our souls. However, there are mothers who don't experience this bond; the connection has been lost or diminished because they are so disconnected from themselves.

Please don't feel guilty if this is hitting home. That is not our goal. We want to relieve you of this burden you're carrying. We want to help you become more satisfied with what you have and who you are, and to help you give up some of the behaviors and attitudes emphasizing what you lack. And that goes far beyond sculpting your body into perfection or losing those last five pounds of postbaby weight.

Any mom of a school-age child will tell you how fast it all goes. The infant days speed by in a blink; the baby and toddler months disappear in a blur. Suddenly, that tiny bundle you stared at in awe has turned into a boisterous dynamo that not only talks, but talks back—or has morphed into a teen complete with eye rolls who insists you stop posting "ILY" on her Facebook wall. You don't want to miss your precious time with your kids worrying about your body and feeling disconnected from your life.

YOUR BODY, YOURSELF

Usually when women think of body image, they think of how they feel about their physical bodies, and how those bodies look. However, body image actually embraces everything about you—not just how you look, but *how you think about yourself as a person*. When Dena works with patients, she describes "body image" as the mental picture you carry of your body, and the thoughts, feelings, and judgments that accompany this image. She breaks it down into three basic components:

- How you see yourself (the picture of yourself in your mind's eye)
- How you *believe* others see you (whether or not this perception is true)
- How you experience living in your body

Body image is impacted by our past experiences, current mood, and feedback from others. Women with positive body image do not define themselves by how they look. They do not tie their self-esteem to their weight on the scale. They know that they are more than their bodies.

Women with poor body image have negative thoughts and feelings about themselves and are unable to view themselves accurately. Their body image is irrevocably linked to their self-esteem. They base their entire identity, purpose, and sense of worth on how they look and how much they weigh.

Ironically, the more attention we pay to dieting, losing weight, and "body checking," the more magnified body image disturbances and body dissatisfaction become. The greater the body disturbance/dissatisfaction, the more disordered a person's eating. And thus, a vicious cycle begins. Three in four women admit that concerns with body size and/or shape interfere with their happiness. Yet it's hard to avoid these concerns in a culture that promotes

- unrealistic expectations of how we're "supposed" to look;
- constant exposure to media images that celebrate unrealistic standards of physical beauty and perfection;
- refusal to accept one's *genetic destiny*—in other words, some women are naturally fleshier, heavier, or curvier than others;
- tying self-esteem to one's physical appearance.

DENA'S STORY

Late Bloomer

When my daughter, Alexis, was three years old, I watched her dance naked in front of the mirror. She was giggling and spinning and feeling free in her body. She was confident, proud, and secure, and I delighted in her joy. But I also distinctly remember feeling sad; one day, the joy she felt over her body and herself might be gone. Would she decide she was "too fat"? Would she follow in my footsteps and be trapped in a food prison for years, obsessing over what she ate and trying to attain a weight that would be impossible to maintain?

I never really thought about what I looked like until I turned sixteen. I was the quintessential "late bloomer." I had a stick-thin body that didn't "develop" until the summer between my sophomore and junior years of high school. When I started my junior year, I had a whole new figure, complete with breasts and hips—and everybody noticed. I had been a cheerleader and dancer before, so I was used to performing in front of people. But this was different. Suddenly all these people (mostly guys, many of whom had never glanced at me before) were paying attention to me. I became one of the most popular girls in school, and while some of the attention felt good, most of it made me very uncomfortable. For the first time, I was truly aware of my body—at least how it looked—and I didn't like it. But I had no time or energy to diet; I was too busy with dance and cheerleading and high school.

It wasn't until my freshman year of college that things got out of control. I had quit dancing and cheerleading, and like many freshmen, had gained weight—about twenty pounds. I was disgusted with myself, and decided to recapture my "normal" body. I tried just about every weight-loss program available back then—Weight Watchers, Jenny Craig, the grapefruit diet, and Jazzercize, to name a few. I'd get up at 4 a.m. to exercise for two and a half hours, starve myself all day while attending classes, and then binge in the dorm cafeteria at dinner. Afterward, I'd force myself to exercise from 9 to 11 p.m. every night. I was exhausted, hungry, irritable, and miserable. I always felt fat, out of control, and "less than." I'd gone from being queen of the class to an environment in which I knew no one. It didn't occur to me that I was really feeling unsure about my identity as a young woman. I just knew I was fat and I had to change it.

Several things happened that shook me up and changed the way I treated my body. My freshman and sophomore years of college, I had two roommates who had anorexia. Seeing the way they starved themselves in their quest for perfection made me realize I didn't want to turn into them. But I also remember thinking, "That's not me. *I'm* not anorexic." And I wasn't—but I hated my body, and I dieted and exercised constantly. Unfortunately, I thought that was normal—until I learned more about psychology, health, and body image.

More Than Looks

Slowly, I began to develop an identity that was more than my body. Continuing with my graduate studies, I valued myself not for what I looked like, but for what I could do. As I started to help others, I found that my obsession with my body's appearance waned. I gradually stopped dieting and punishing myself with hours of exercise. My weight normalized because I wasn't trying to control it.

In the meantime, my roommates with anorexia continued to struggle. One sought treatment and eventually recovered. The other, Andrea, died of heart failure at the age of twenty-four. That incident broke me and convinced me to specialize in eating disorders. After all, I'd already seen the devastation they could cause. In my late twenties, I accepted my body by abandoning the idea of changing or molding it. Soon afterward, I met my husband and got married, while continuing to work with women with eating disorders. My life had reached a comfortable, happy stasis.

Baby Weight

Then I became a mom. I gained sixty pounds with my first pregnancy, more than twice what I "should" have. By my third trimester, I started turning around on the scale at my doctor's office so I wouldn't see the number. I was thrilled to be carrying a baby and excited to become a mother, but I sure didn't compare to the beautiful pregnant celebrities sporting tiny "baby bumps," designer maternity clothes, and four-inch heels. I would never have said this to my patients, but I didn't feel beautiful. I felt fat and disgusting. And anyone who says "fat is not a feeling" doesn't know anything about being a woman in this country. Once Alexis arrived, I was so busy (and overwhelmed) that I didn't worry about the extra weight right away—but I started experiencing that too-familiar feeling of being uncomfortable in my own skin.

It wasn't until after having my son, Erik, that I was able to reach a stable, healthy weight—and this didn't happen by dieting or hating my larger, somewhat softer body. Instead, I decided to follow the advice I'd been giving patients for years: to use balance, variety, and moderation in my approach to food, and to take care of my body through regular exercise. This allowed me to accept my "new" body.

MOM FIRST, WOMAN SECOND?

You already know that you're one of the most influential role models your children have, whether you want to be or not. A study conducted in Australia examined the impact parents have on the body image of teens. Researchers found that although both parents matter, mothers have a larger impact on weight-related issues because they tend to diet more, play a greater role in food preparation, and generally address issues surrounding food and weight.

Another study of younger children, aged seven through ten, found that the more they felt their mothers wanted them to be thin, the more dissatisfied they were with their own bodies—and the more likely to report unhealthy weight control behaviors. In addition, children who thought their mothers were worried about their own weight also tended to restrict.

We're sure you know that when parents have issues with *anything*—whether it's alcohol, violence, or poor money management—their feelings affect their children. And it's fine to improve the way you treat yourself in order to be a better role model for your children; most moms think of themselves as a mother first, woman second. But tending to the *woman* in you will also benefit you as a mother. In the end, it doesn't matter whether you're motivated by your children or by yourself; the benefits of addressing your body image and eating issues will bless both you and those you love.

We also want to speak to the women reading this who are thinking, "I hear what you're saying, and you're probably right, but I really *am* too fat! I need to lose weight first! *Then* I'll have better eating habits and a better body image." If you're so heavy you can't get out of a chair, or you have health problems related to your weight, then yes, you'd benefit from dropping some pounds. But the answer isn't to go on a diet. It's to change both your lifestyle and your attitude—not only toward food, but toward yourself. When you feel good about your body—even if it's not the perfect one sold by media—you'll find it's easier to treat yourself with kindness, respect, and even love. We've seen it firsthand with hundreds of women.

It's not easy. Overcoming years of disordered eating, terrible body image, and using yourself as your own punching bag takes focus, hard work, and determination. But it *can* be done. We've seen women who were caught up in a cycle of self-hate and starving learn to eat normally and live healthier, happier lives. We've seen women who binged and purged day after day learn how to treat food like fuel for their bodies, not as a way of managing uncomfortable emotions. And we've seen women who were completely disconnected from themselves and their families learn how to reconnect, to appreciate and accept their bodies, and to dote on their children and husbands. So don't despair. Whoever you are, wherever you're at, it's never too late to learn how to love.

REFLECTION

Of course every woman is different. Some women are fortunate to have a secure, positive body image and an uncomplicated relationship with food. (Hard to believe, isn't it?) If you're in the majority, though, you find it hard to love yourself and to eat healthily. Take this quiz to get a better handle on your relationship with your body, your soul, and your appetite.

1. If you suddenly gained five pounds, you'd feel:
   a. Sick with dread.
   b. Worried and stressed out—what if you gain even more weight?

    c. Uncomfortable.

    d. Okay—and realize you've been eating more or exercising less.

2. How often do you diet or otherwise limit what you eat?

    a. All the time.

    b. Every Monday—though I usually fall off the diet by Friday.

    c. Occasionally.

    d. Once in a while.

3. How often do you criticize your body (out loud or not)?

    a. Constantly.

    b. Every day.

    c. When I go shopping and can't fit into something I like.

    d. Once in a while.

4. What's your *primary* reason for exercising?

    a. To lose weight.

    b. To stay thin.

    c. To reduce stress.

    d. To be healthy.

5. Have you ever exercised when you've been sick or injured?

    a. Yes—I never miss a workout.

    b. Sure, or I will gain weight.

    c. Once in a while, depending on how stressed out I feel.

    d. Nope—that would just make me feel worse.

6. Do you ever purge (whether by vomiting, taking laxatives, or exercising excessively) to get rid of calories?

    a. Yes, at least several times a month.

    b. Yes, if I have overeaten.

    c. I have in the past but am not doing it now.

    d. Never.

7. Do you feel like your eating is out of control?

    a. Yes!

    b. Often—I have a hard time limiting what I eat.

    c. Occasionally, especially when I'm socializing.

    d. No, I stay in balance.

8. How often do you think about food or about what you'll be eating next?

a. All the time.

b. At least half the time.

c. Fairly often.

d. I think about it when I'm hungry or planning a meal.

9. Do you ever worry about your child's eating habits or body size/shape?

   a. Yes, all the time. I don't want him or her to be fat!

   b. Yes, because I know how hard it is to lose weight as an adult.

   c. Yes, because I worry about how much junk food he or she eats.

   d. Yes, because I want him or her to be healthy.

10. If your child is/became overweight, how do/would you feel?

    a. Horrible—like I failed as a parent.

    b. Really upset—I don't want him or her to feel bad.

    c. Worried that he or she will grow into an overweight adult.

    d. Worried that he or she isn't healthy, and isn't getting enough activity.

11. Have you ever tried to lose weight by eating a low-calorie restrictive diet?

    a. Yes, at least twenty times.

    b. Frequently, at least ten times.

    c. Occasionally.

    d. Seldom.

12. Do you often dress to hide your "flaws"?

    a. All the time.

    b. It depends on how I look that day, or whether I've gained weight.

    c. Sometimes.

    d. I don't really think about it.

13. Do you ever compare your body to others—whether to celebrities' or friends'?

    a. All the time—and mine never measures up.

    b. Sure—who doesn't?

    c. Sometimes, but I realize that everyone's body is different.

    d. Seldom.

14. Do you worry about controlling how much, or what kinds of foods, you're eating?
    a. Yes—I can't have certain foods in the house.
    b. Yes—I'm very careful about my portions.
    c. Occasionally, if I notice I've gained weight.
    d. Very seldom.
15. How often does physical hunger dictate whether you eat?
    a. Never—I eat according to what my diet says.
    b. I try not to eat until I can't stand my hunger anymore.
    c. It depends on how hungry I am and what I have at hand.
    d. When I'm hungry, I eat to refuel my body.
16. How often do you eat what you want to eat?
    a. Never.
    b. Very rarely.
    c. Sometimes.
    d. Most of the time.
17. How often do you weigh yourself?
    a. Several times a day.
    b. Every morning.
    c. Once or twice a week.
    d. Once in a while—or at my annual checkup.
18. Have your kids ever heard you say something negative about your body?
    a. Yes—all the time.
    b. Frequently, although I try not to say negative things in front of them.
    c. Once in a while.
    d. I don't think so.
19. How often do you eat the same food as your children?
    a. Never—I'm always dieting.
    b. Rarely—I make food for them and something else for myself.
    c. Occasionally.
    d. Most of the time.
20. Let's say you were just told that "this is it—your body shape will *never* change regardless of how hard you try." How do you feel?

a. Devastated—I can't imagine not being thinner.
b. Disappointed that I'm "stuck" in this body for the rest of my life.
c. Relieved that I don't have to think about dieting anymore.
d. Content.

How did you do? Give yourself four points for each *a* answer, three points for every *b*, two points for each *c*, and one point for every *d*. Obviously, this quiz isn't meant to be an extensive analysis of your possible food and body image issues, but the higher your score, the more you may be struggling with your body image, eating habits, and your sense of yourself as a woman—and the more you may need this book. A score greater than 60 indicates you may have a lot of food and body image issues; 30 to 59 suggests that you're more of the "average" woman; and a score of less than 30 indicates that you're one of the few women who retain a confident sense of self. Good for you!

A Special Note for High Scorers

Scoring high on this quiz isn't a good thing. If you scored more than 60, you may also want to take this simple "SCOFF" test that is used to identify eating disorders:

1. Do you make yourself **S**ick because you feel uncomfortably full?
2. Do you worry that you have lost **C**ontrol over how much you eat?
3. Have you recently lost more than **O**ne stone (fourteen pounds) in a three-month period (not including postpartum weight loss or other medical scenarios)?
4. Do you believe yourself to be **F**at when others say you are too thin?
5. Would you say that **F**ood dominates your life?

Give yourself a point for every "yes" answer. A score of 2 or more indicates a likely case of anorexia or bulimia, and you may benefit from seeking professional help. Most women with eating disorders cannot recover on their own, so please don't feel guilty or ashamed about reaching out for help or support. (You'll find a list of resources at the back of this book.)

TOOLS

Take some time to journal about your relationship with food, yourself, your husband, and your children. Write down the predominant emotions you experience when it comes to each: fear, shame, guilt, joy, happiness, excitement, and so on. Then, consider how you hope to grow or change in each area, and write down specific goals. Be courageous and bold; this is your life.

A Bruised Beginning

From Girlhood to Adolescence

It is never too late to have a happy childhood.

—Tom Robbins

As girls, we pretend to be princesses. We put on pink dresses and throw back our golden locks and wait for our knights in shining armor to whisk us away on noble steeds. And some of us play mother-and-child, pushing dollies in carriages and dressing cats in frilly bonnets and pretending to nurse; we dream of the day when we'll have ten children and be adored by a man, and it all seems so magical.

Until we get boobs and hips and hormones. Until boys and men start noticing us—perhaps too closely—and we're forced to grow up in very painful ways. We abandon all hopes of being princesses and instead, long to hide.

Then there are the rest of us, on the other side of the spectrum, with flat chests and braces and we *are* invisible. We long to be noticed, and there's no joy in pretending. There's only someone's daughter in loose-fit clothing. "This is when girls learn to be nice rather than honest," writes Mary Pipher.[1]

This is also when we lose ourselves. It is when we go into hiding, trying to escape a world we no longer know, a world with too many eyes and too few princes, a world that aches for salvation. As Pipher puts it, "Young girls slowly bury their childhood, put away their independent and imperious selves and submissively enter adult existence."[2]

And this is when the cycle of self-abuse begins. It is a cycle that, for most women, continues long into adulthood. Some girls simply quietly despise themselves, perhaps because of a negative home environment— their fathers put them down, their uncles sexually molest them, their mothers look the other way. Or perhaps the stress happens outside the home: they're bullied at school, or raped by a teacher, or they experience trauma of some other sort. So they wear frumpy clothes and try to look in the mirror as little as possible, and they talk negatively about themselves.

And then there are those who go to the extreme and develop eating disorders.

THE CRIES OF A CHILD

Lisa was skin and bones on the couch in the basement. She was a slip of a thing at twelve years old, and her eyes seemed like empty plates. She was watching TV, and nothing was working, her parents said. They couldn't get her to eat.

Being mothers ourselves, we wanted to reach out. So we'd come to hear this little girl's story. To hear why she'd been starving herself since the age of seven. *Seven.* Grade two. When other little girls were playing tag at recess and braiding each other's hair and throwing crayons at boys, Lisa was throwing away her lunch and sucking in her stomach.

She told us it was because her daddy had gone on a diet. This was an innocent enough gesture on his part, but he was her hero. She was "Daddy's little girl," and she hung on his words and saw the way he scorned his body. He made fun of his fat and called other people *big* or *overweight*. And she wanted to be beautiful in her daddy's eyes, so she'd gone on a diet too.

Yet, while his diet had ended after a few weeks, hers had developed into a mental illness, now five years and counting. It had become a lifestyle, a disordered way of eating, a disordered way of viewing herself and the world. It was a diet that had turned into self-abuse—into overexercise and serious starvation. For hours each night, this little girl did crunches and ran laps in her room. She weighed herself after every meal, after every washroom break, and after every bath—standing naked and smiling at the way the numbers dropped when she wore no clothes. It was a diet that had taken over Lisa's schoolwork, her grades dropping like her weight because she couldn't focus in class and she went to bed at seven, too tired to stay awake. And she looked like she was sleeping now: even while she was talking to us, like her whole face had gone on vacation.

She was tortured, this girl, and while it might seem strange—deliberately making choices that caused her to be unhappy—we understood. Even after having two beautiful children each, we knew how easy it was to fall back into disordered eating, how tempting the destructive lifestyle was. It makes a person feel like she is in control, and motherhood is perhaps one of the most uncontrollable processes we'll ever experience.

A World Vision commercial came on as we sat there with this young girl. She turned and stared at the screen. A little African boy with bony arms and ribs stared back at her while a voice begged people to donate. Lisa turned to us and said, "That kid is so lucky. He doesn't have to eat."

Anne Lamott writes, "This culture's pursuit of beauty is a crazy, sick, losing game, for women, men, teenagers, and with the need to increase advertising revenues, now for pre-adolescents, too. We're starting to see more and more anorexic eight- and-nine-year-olds. It's a game we cannot win. Every time we agree to play another round, and step out onto the court to try again, we've already lost. The only way to win is to stay off the court. . . . Lies cannot nourish or protect you. Only freedom from fear, freedom from lies, can make us beautiful, and keep us safe."[3]

DEFINING THE DISORDERS

In some ways, we all struggle with disordered eating. Most of us, at some point or another, skip a meal or go on a diet or consume too much chocolate (and not enough vegetables). We stuff ourselves at buffets and eat nothing for breakfast, and we know what it's like to feel bloated or sick from having mistreated our hunger cues. But then there are those who take it further, those whose attempts to gain control over their size and their lives turns into a compulsion. The eating disorder becomes an alternate identity, a way to deal with abuse and neglect, a way to feel normal, or a subconscious means of escaping this world altogether.

According to the Mayo Clinic, "Eating disorders are a group of serious conditions in which you're so preoccupied with food and weight that you can often focus on little else."[4] There is no set cause for these conditions. The obsession our culture has with thinness, youth, and beauty contributes to their development; however, genetic vulnerability, personality traits, and psychological and environmental factors also play a part. An eating disorder (namely, anorexia nervosa, bulimia nervosa, and binge eating disorder) is a condition that meets criteria outlined in the *DSM-IV*, the *Diagnostic and Statistical Manual of Mental Disorders, Fourth Edition*.

Anorexia nervosa, commonly called *anorexia*, affects between 1 and 4 percent of American females at some point during their lives. *DSM-IV* criteria include:

a. Refusal to maintain body weight at or above a minimally normal weight for age and height (e.g., weight loss leading to maintenance of body weight less than 85 percent of that expected; or failure to make expected weight gain during period of growth, leading to body weight less than 85 percent of that expected)
b. Intense fear of gaining weight or becoming fat, even though underweight
c. Disturbance over the way one's body weight or shape is experienced; undue influence of body shape on self-evaluation, or denial of the seriousness of the current low body weight
d. In postmenarcheal females, amenorrhea, that is, the absence of at least three consecutive menstrual cycles

Bulimia nervosa, referred to as *bulimia*, affects 1–5 percent of the population. Criteria consist of:

  a. Recurrent episodes of binge eating, such as
    i Eating, in a discrete period of time (e.g., within any two-hour period), an amount of food that is definitely larger than what most people would eat during a similar period of time and under similar circumstances
    ii. A sense of lack of control over eating during the episode (e.g., a feeling that one cannot stop eating or control what or how much one is eating)
  b. Recurrent inappropriate compensatory behavior in order to prevent weight gain, such as self-induced vomiting, misuse of laxatives, diuretics, enemas, or other medications; fasting; or excessive exercise
  c. The binge eating and inappropriate compensatory behaviors occur, on average, at least twice a week for three months
  d. Self-evaluation is unduly influenced by body shape and weight
  e. The disturbance does not occur exclusively during episodes of anorexia nervosa

Stress turns into dieting, which turns into starvation or bingeing and purging, which turns into a mental illness, and it's often underlined by genetics. According to the website Something Fishy, "One study by doctors at the Maudsley Hospital in London suggested that people with anorexia were twice as likely to have variations in the gene for serotonin receptors, part of which helps to determine appetite."[5] This overproduction of serotonin creates a sensation of extreme stress—causing overwhelming and constant anxiety—which in turn triggers anorexia.[6]

A study conducted by Dr. Walter Kaye, program director of the Eating Disorders Program at the University of California, San Diego, School of Medicine, examined a number of recovered bulimia patients, monitoring them for persistent behavior disturbances and levels of serotonin, dopamine, and norepinephrine. Results showed that, compared to those with no history of bulimia, the recovered individuals still exhibited unusual serotonin levels, with more negative moods, and obsessions with perfectionism and exactness. The levels of the other brain chemicals, dopamine and norepinephrine, were normal in comparison.[7]

The primary "clinical" eating disorders represent about ten to fourteen million American women. "Well, that's not me," you may be thinking. "*I* don't have an eating disorder!" You may not, but you're probably one of the tens of millions of women who struggle with disordered eating and poor body image. "On any given day, nearly 40 percent of American women are on a diet," writes Jenny Deam in a recent *Women's Health* article. "The weight-worry gun is loaded early: By the time they reach age 10, 80 percent of girls fret that they're fat. Their main 'thinspiration,' according to experts: the ultra-slim starlets glorified in popular culture."[8]

If you deny yourself food when you're hungry; if you're constantly trying to lose weight by slashing calories; if you're afraid to eat certain foods or beat yourself up when you do; if you're constantly obsessing over food, you may be like most other women, but that's not "normal," even if it seems to be. In fact, you may have what has been defined as an "eating disorder not otherwise specified" (EDNOS). This includes emotional/stress eating, binge eating, chronic dieting, restrictive eating, and purging, as well as some newly defined disorders: orthorexia—a fixation with healthy or righteous eating; pregorexia—extreme dieting and exercising while pregnant to avoid gaining the twenty-five to thirty-five pounds of weight doctors usually recommend; anorexia athletica—an addiction to exercise; drunkorexia—restricting food intake in order to reserve those calories for alcohol and binge drinking; and diabulimia—in which those with type 1 diabetes deliberately restrict their insulin intake for the purpose of weight loss.[9]

The *DSM-IV* definition for EDNOS implies that

- all the criteria for anorexia nervosa are met except that the individual has regular menses;
- all the criteria for anorexia nervosa are met except that, despite substantial weight loss, the individual's current weight is in the normal range;
- all the criteria for bulimia nervosa are met except that binges occur at a frequency of less than twice a week or for a period of less than three months;
- an individual of normal body weight regularly engages in inappropriate compensatory behavior after eating small amounts of

food (e.g., self-induced vomiting after the consumption of two cookies);

- an individual repeatedly chews and spits out, but does not swallow, large amounts of food.[10]

Society breeds a distorted perspective of self through its magazines and billboards. Women are taught that anxiety over food and weight is normal, and expected, while men are often encouraged to self-indulge. As a result, none of us is truly free. We're all trapped in adolescence, trying to fit in with the cool crowd. Disordered eating is merely a manifestation of our discontent with ourselves.

REDEFINING OURSELVES

Even the most confident of women is going to have bad days—days in which she looks in the mirror and groans. *But those bad days don't need to define us.*

Miranda is a nurse and a mother of three who's never had an eating disorder. But she still struggles with her reflection. She still has days when she wears sweats so she doesn't have to feel her pants getting tighter. "If I am having a 'bad' day, I usually think things like, 'Ugh, I don't want to get all dressed up and go out,'" she says.

When it comes to dealing with those thoughts, Miranda admits that if she tries to make herself look good by putting on makeup and nice earrings, she generally feels better, "so it is more just about making the effort, and the feeling follows." But when that doesn't work, she says, she gives herself pep talks, as in, "'Think about how lucky you are to have these wonderful healthy children! Who cares about your pants?'"

When Emily's youngest sister had her baby, Emily went to visit. She noticed a bottle of stretch-mark lotion in the bathroom, and her sister asked how long it would take before it made the marks disappear.

"I don't know," said Emily. "I've never used the cream." Then she took her little sister's shoulders in her hands and looked her in the eyes and said gently, "These are our beauty marks. Our war wounds. We need to wear them proudly. To declare to the world, 'Look! I've given life—and I've got proof!'"

And then there's food—beautiful, sensual, delectable food that we, in North America, are fortunate to have in abundance. We cannot live without it; we are born needing it, and as pregnant women, our daily intake provides nutrients for the life growing within. When our children emerge from the womb, we continue to feed them, to nourish with milk produced by our bodies, and a baby's slurps and gurgles prove how delightful food can be. As Emily's husband, a farmer's son, says, "Food is a celebration—a gift from God to be enjoyed."

Why, then, is it so complicated? When does it get confusing? And how do we make it simple again?

EMILY'S STORY

How I Became Anorexic

Food became hard for me when I was just nine years old. Well, actually, life became hard for me—too hard for tears to fix. My Grandma Ermenie had just died. Up until that point, I hadn't realized God would let you get close to someone only to take her away. I hadn't realized how final death was. And I had no one to talk to about it.

My mother was a British woman, very quiet and demure and self-conscious, who blushed when Dad tried to kiss her in public. She didn't like to talk about anything to do with the body, and wouldn't let us play with Barbie dolls or take dance lessons or look at fashion magazines. She homeschooled us—me until I was in grade five—and was overworked and underappreciated, and didn't have the mental or emotional strength to let us know, verbally, how valuable we were. All of this stemmed from Mum's never having known how valuable *she* was. Her mum (my Nanny) had longed to be an artist, and had openly regretted the fact that she'd had children. My mother doesn't remember Nanny ever saying, "I love you."

And my dad, while a kind, godly man, didn't help matters. He had been raised on a dairy farm with two brothers and a father who believed that women, like my humble, quiet grandmother, were to be seen, not heard. My father spent many years putting ministry before family. He was always gone on some clergy call or another, and by the time he got home he was too tired to put much effort into matters that he figured were my mother's domain. So he tended toward authoritarianism, and I grew up despising authority because to me, it meant a distant character who was never around long enough to get to know me.

While both my parents had perfectly good reasons for being the people they were, I grew up feeling unloved and unwanted. It wasn't that my parents didn't provide for me; there just wasn't a lot of heart in it. For some kids, this wouldn't have mattered, but I was a sensitive, aesthetic, needy child. Add to that the fact that we moved 10 times in seven years, and you have the case for why I stopped eating after Grandma Ermenie died. I'd resolved to never feel pain again. Some people use eating as a drug. They overconsume until they feel numb. I used starvation. Both methods serve the same purpose.

For me as a nine-year-old, everything had to be tiny. For some reason, tiny meant perfect because society told me thin was beauty. So even my writing turned small, and my teachers complained that their eyes hurt, but there was safety in the little blue letters lined up neat.

Eventually the label on my jeans said size 0 and I knew I'd gotten as little as I could without disappearing altogether. I wrote small until I had nothing left to say. And then I waited to feel good. I waited to feel the way perfection is meant to feel. I waited to feel the love the world told me that skinny would earn. But all I got was admitted into a hospital.

STARVING FOR LOVE

I grew up with an abnormal desire to please everyone and discovered that no one is ever pleased all the time, so I stopped eating because everyone's disappointment hurt too much. We were to be seen and not heard. I didn't say anything. I just starved myself. It was my way of being heard.

I believe that we, as humans, are created to desire perfection, for God is perfect, but not in the way that some churches and homeschooling families seem to dictate. Perfection is not something that can be earned. It is grace, bestowed. It is not a behavior or a set of rules. Rather, it is a gift.

I didn't love myself, and even after years of losing weight, this thirteen-year-old could only look in the mirror and cry; no amount of eating or not eating can resolve something food isn't intended to fill. No amount of the physical can satisfy the spiritual.

I started to eat again, finally, because I knew that otherwise I would die. The nurses couldn't believe I was still alive, and my parents told me I was a miracle, but it would take another thirteen years, another relapse into anorexia, and a sacrificial husband before I'd believe it myself.

REFLECTION

- What are your bruises? When did they form, and how do they continue to hurt?
- Whom do you subconsciously, or consciously, blame for your war wounds? Are you open to the idea of forgiving them?
- How does your bruised soul affect the way you mother your children?
- How do you take your disappointments out on food?
- What kinds of unmet needs are you still trying to have your family fill?

TOOLS

- Every morning when you get out of bed, practice telling yourself that you are beautifully and wonderfully made.
- Consider your gifts and what your spiritual identity (your unique calling) might be. Ask friends and family members to help you in this area, to discern your strengths and to help you know what you're good at.
- Make a list of needs that weren't met for you as a child; consider releasing those needs and forgiving the people who didn't meet them, so you, in turn, might be free.

From Bruised to Broken

When Adolescent Turns Adult

There is in every true woman's heart, a spark of heavenly fire, which lies dormant in the broad daylight of prosperity, but which kindles up and beams and blazes in the dark hour of adversity.

—Washington Irving

Bruised girls thus become confused adolescents and then paranoid women who try to appease society, knowing all the while they were made for more—more than sucking in their stomachs and counting calories and worrying about how their butt looks in a pair of jeans. And yes, it is normal to be disappointed in ourselves, to sometimes regret the reflection staring back at us. It doesn't mean we have an eating disorder. But it probably means we're discontent with our body image, when shouldn't we be kinder to ourselves? More loving?

The problem is that we, as women, haven't been encouraged to love ourselves because that wouldn't feed the cosmetics industry. So, our bruises remain hidden beneath layers of cover-up, and we step into womanhood, beaten down and searching for someone to make us feel better about ourselves. But unless we remove the makeup and allow our bruises to heal, we'll never feel better.

We get married anyway, and there's nothing magical about two broken people vowing to love each other for better or worse. It's crazy hard, and some days, it feels impossible. You don't know who you are, and you despise the person you think you are, and then you marry someone who claims to adore you, and you become convinced he is lying because who can really love you? You don't even love yourself. This is not exactly a strong premise for marriage. So the broken woman becomes a broken wife with a shattered reflection.

A SLOW JOURNEY

Marriage is all about sharing. But when you don't know who you are, or you don't like who you are, it's hard to share yourself with someone else. So, many of us who have struggled with eating issues and body image problems don't. Instead, we clam up and shut down until the people who believe in us realize they actually don't know us. And then they walk away.

It doesn't have to be this way. It is possible to find the courage to be real and, in turn, to love the real. But healing doesn't happen overnight. We (Emily and Dena) still struggle with wanting to be people who we're not—some days more than others. Because we have restricted our food intake for years, things like portion size and recognizing the body's satiety cues don't come naturally.

Slowly, however, we are learning our triggers. We are learning that stress, and change, and uncontrollable situations make us want to latch onto dieting and disordered eating like a lifeboat. It's important for anyone who struggles with disordered body image or eating habits to learn what triggers this mind-set, the feelings that cause one to enter that dark place. And once you recognize those triggers, it is important to find accountability partners—people who love you enough to tell you when you're wrong, who love you enough to point out the lies, and to reorient you toward the truth.

Physical symptoms such as sleeplessness, irritability, and depression often indicate something is wrong internally—that we need to take better care of ourselves by tending to those inner places, by doing fewer activities, eating more nutritiously, and praying more often. But we'll only start to take better care of ourselves upon realizing that we deserve love—not for any reason other than the fact that we are alive, and *this* makes us valuable. It has nothing to do with being a good mom or wife or a beautiful woman. It has nothing to do with *us* at all. It has everything to do with God's desiring our existence.

We are not accidents. No matter the circumstances that brought us into this world, we are more than our names, more than our roles, more than our dress sizes. We are very intentionally planned creations, and we have a spiritual purpose here on earth. This knowing that *I am more than what I see in the mirror* can help us, every day, to treat ourselves with love.

HOW TO LET HEALING HAPPEN

So how do we let our needs, our spiritual bruises, be healed by an invisible being? By a divine person we cannot see? How do we experience spiritual love and let it soothe our wounds?

"Do we believe that it was a power of love which created everything and saw it was good?" writes Madeleine L'Engle. "Is creation purposeful? Or is it some kind of cosmic accident? Do our fragments of lives have meaning? . . . Can we see the pattern and beauty which is an affirmation of the value of all creation?"[1]

Love begins with a belief in something higher, something better than us. Then, it requires repentance: acknowledging the mess-ups we are, and the mystery God is, and the way he reached down to save us from ourselves. It requires us to accept God's forgiveness, and then to forgive ourselves, and finally, to forgive all of those who have hurt us in the past. This is hard but extremely worthwhile because forgiveness is the doorway to joy. As William Paul Young writes in *The Shack*, "Forgiveness is not about forgetting. It is about letting go of another person's throat. . . . Forgiveness does not create a relationship. Unless people speak the truth about what they have done and change their mind and behavior, a relationship of trust is not possible. When you forgive someone you certainly release them from judgment, but without true change, no real relationship can be established. . . . Forgiveness in no way requires that you trust the one you forgive. But should they finally confess and repent, you will discover a miracle in your own heart that allows you to reach out and begin to build between you a bridge of reconciliation. . . . Forgiveness does not excuse anything. . . . You may have to declare your forgiveness a hundred times the first day and the second day, but the third day will be less and each day after, until one day you will realize that you have forgiven completely. And then one day you will pray for his wholeness."[2]

Last, love requires hope, hope that God will reveal the extent of his love for us, that we "may have power, together with all of the Lord's holy people, to grasp how wide and long and high and deep is the love of Christ, and to know this love that surpasses knowledge—that [we] may be filled to the measure of all the fullness of God" (Ephesians 3:17–19). Even if you don't share the Christian faith, it is still possible to believe you were made for something more, something greater than a disordered eating lifestyle.

"It's strange to be an American female because, from the age of about four, you're taught your value lies in being adorable and entertaining and very female," writes Anne Lamott. "So my body has gotten bigger and older . . . and I wish I'd worn sunscreen and turtlenecks . . . but when I am able to extend grace to myself, there is an absolute change in my feeling about the rest of the world.

"I put a lot of lotion on . . . my legs. Sometimes I put on one of those Band-Aids that kids use, like a rose tattoo . . . and I'm kind with myself and talk to myself as I would with a close friend. I say, 'You are so strong . . . your legs are so sturdy, they're just beautiful. . . .' Let's just be in gratitude, instead of the anxiety that I don't look like Cameron Diaz. Cameron Diaz doesn't even look like Cameron Diaz."[3]

FINDING A NEW IDENTITY

Emily's Story

It was July and the sun was searing hot and I was getting married in the backyard of my parents' home. I wore vines wound around my head and my dress was empire waist. I had five bridesmaids who wore different colored dresses. They looked like poppies swaying in the slight breeze.

Trent and his groomsmen were sweating in black suits. I was sweating too, but it wasn't from the sun.

My dad was the pastor marrying us beneath a trellis climbing with roses. "I now pronounce you man and wife," he said. Trent kissed me and I gripped my basket of petals until my knuckles turned white. It would be weeks until my husband realized he'd married a woman he no longer knew.

I'd been in recovery from anorexia for ten years. When Trent met me at Bible School, I was a straw-haired hippie high on life. We dated on and off, and then one day when he was sick with a migraine, he asked me if I would take care of him forever, and I said yes. He knew about my past; he knew about the eating disorder, but he was a boy from a farm. He'd grown up growing food, and so food was a natural part of life, not something to be deleted or calculated or measured, and he didn't understand starvation and I didn't need him to. I was over it, I said.

After we got engaged, I went to the Middle East for six months. While I was there, I put on weight, for every time I entered someone's home, I was served platters of fruit and sweets. I couldn't say no, for that would have been rude, and I didn't notice my pants becoming snug. That is, not until the day I was eating a sandwich and a Lebanese friend of mine said in Arabic, "You've put on weight." I immediately dropped the sandwich and everything flooded back: the shame, the guilt, the despair of never being good enough that had led to my eating disorder in the first place. I'm not sure what it is about women and guilt, but I was born feeling it: feeling responsible for the world and its problems, as though I am somehow to blame. And when you have children, the guilt only intensifies.

But the young woman who returned from Lebanon didn't want children anymore—having children would have meant getting pregnant, and getting pregnant meant gaining weight. No, I had a new mission. I was going to get skinny, and nothing would distract me this time. Not even my soon-to-be husband.

My anxiety over my weight only intensified when I got married. As a wife, I no longer knew who I was. All I'd ever really had—all that had ever really stayed constant in a childhood of transition and upheaval—was my name. I was *Emily Dow*. And then suddenly, that was gone, too. I became "Mrs. Wierenga," and that meant nothing to me, only that I belonged to someone else. So when my father said, "It is my pleasure to introduce you to Mr. and Mrs. Wierenga" and the crowd rose from its fold-up chairs and applauded as Trent and I walked down the aisle, I felt the lid closing down on what had been my life.

"I knew something was really wrong when you didn't want butter on your popcorn," my husband recalls.

We'd been living together for a few months in the basement of a friend's house, and Trent had planned a date night. He'd rented a movie and made popcorn, and I had panicked when I'd seen the butter he'd put on the popcorn. I'd cried and yelled and insisted on making my own bowl. Then I'd sprinkled salt onto the kernels and the salt had fallen to the bottom of the dish, with nothing to hold on to.

The anorexic relapse had begun slowly, with the dropping of the sandwich, but quickly accelerated into nine cups of coffee a day and nothing for breakfast or lunch. I would overeat at supper, trying to fill myself up for the following day, when the starvation would start all over again. The difference between the relapse and the original eating disorder was that this time I knew what I was doing. I knew I was starving myself. And I was okay with it because at least I didn't have to deal with all the questions, questions like, "Who am I?" and "Who is he?" and "Why did I ever get married?"

Eventually, though, the questions caught up with me. Eventually, Trent stopped being patient and started getting worried that I was going to die. And one day, as we were driving down the highway and screaming at each other, and I tried to drive into oncoming traffic, Trent took the steering wheel and pulled over to the side of the road. Then he gave me an ultimatum. It was him or food. After a long pause, I chose him. When Trent gave me that ultimatum, he made me believe I was worth something. He was willing to sacrifice his happiness for my health. He was willing to lay it all on the line so that I could get better, and this told me that I was special.

And isn't this all we ever want? From the moment we're born, until the day we die, don't we all just want to know that we're valuable? That our living here on this earth among millions of other people means something? So I found meaning in his eyes that day on the highway. I found meaning in his act of sacrificial love, and I discovered a new mission: to live for others—first, my husband, and later on, my children. I wasn't being asked to lose myself, in order to become wife or mother. Instead, I was being challenged to find those role(s) within myself, to uncover some of the gifts that had been embedded in me, as a female, when I was conceived, to allow them to develop and flourish. Instead of losing myself, I was becoming more of myself.

"It's funny," writes Lamott. "I always imagined when I was a kid that adults had some kind of inner toolbox full of shiny tools: the saw of discernment, the hammer of wisdom, the sandpaper of patience. But then when I grew up, I found that life handed you these rusty bent old tools—friendships, prayer, conscience, honesty—and said 'do the best you can with these, they will have to do.' And mostly, against all odds, they do."[4]

So I began to do the best I could with what I'd been given, and over time, as I studied menus and forgave my parents and realized I was more than the sum of the parts of my life—that I was, in fact, infinitely more valuable than I could ever dream or imagine, and that God was terribly in love with me—those rusty old tools became shiny and new.

REFLECTION

- How emotionally bruised were you when you got married?
- Do you look to your husband to fix your problems, or do you blame him for them?
- How healthy was your self-esteem when you became an adult?
- How did it change when you got married?
- Do you feel like you know who you are?
- Do you believe your husband when he tells you you're beautiful? Why or why not?
- Do you tend to despise or accept your reflection?
- Do you believe you can ever be free of self-hate? Why or why not?

TOOLS

- Look at some old photos of yourself as a little girl, and then some as a young married woman. Then compare those with some current photos; what do you see? In which pictures do you look happiest? Why do you think this is?

- Make a list of personality traits that define who you are now, and compare them with the traits you had as a little girl. How have they changed?
- Spend a night talking to your husband about when you first met, and ask him to remind you of what first attracted him to you. Focus on the love in his eyes, and consider why you find it hard to believe that you are lovable.

BEFORE AND AFTER

The Effects of Pregnancy

Everything grows rounder and wider and weirder, and I sit here in the middle of it all and wonder who in the world you will turn out to be.

—Carrie Fisher

Women are made to give birth, and only women can do it. But just because it comes naturally doesn't mean it's easy. Some women *do* breeze through pregnancy and labor. Most, however, struggle with restless legs and back pain, morning sickness and a perpetual look of confusion that says, "Why am I doing this again?" This is interrupted by the magical flutter of little feet against the insides of their womb. And then, labor, contractions, ear-piercing screams, and tearing.

For a moment, there's bliss, as they hold onto that precious life and look into eyes that remind them of their grandmother's. This is followed by breast-feeding and colic, lack of sleep and spit-up. Add to this the roller-coaster of hormones, the deflated belly, the desire to lose the weight gained during pregnancy, and you have a recipe for low self-esteem.

Even if you've never struggled with disordered eating, it's hard to know how to eat during pregnancy and breast-feeding for optimal health, how to get those extra calories while remaining in shape, and how to lose weight afterward while providing nourishment to another human being if you choose to breast-feed. During pregnancy, you're expanding and bloated and there's someone kicking you from the inside. Everyone wants to touch your tummy, and suddenly, you've lost the rights to your own body. Then the baby emerges and latches on, and you still have marital duties to perform, and possibly other children to care for, not to mention postpartum depression to deal with and maybe a job to return to. As Anne Lamott writes, "I'm going to have an awards banquet for my body when all of this is over."[1]

But until it's over, how does one do it? How does one cope with these physical and emotional changes while handling the pressures of everyday life?

Brandee recalls a moment that gave her hope, even as she sat nursing her newborn. "I'm very large-breasted," she writes.[2] "Forty DD. For the most part, it hasn't bothered me, but—because my breasts are bigger—they're not exactly perky.

"Anyway, the most wonderful thing happened to me after one of the girls was born. I was breastfeeding in the hospital bed, and a young nurse walked in and looked directly at my exposed breast and my infant daughter, nursing there. And she said: 'Wow. That is the most amazing breastfeeding breast I've ever seen.' And it's true: I have amazing, breastfeeding breasts. My nipples are like pencil erasers: very easy for a baby to grasp.

"And it was, honestly, one of the most beautiful and important things anyone has ever said about my body. I felt so proud in that instant, knowing she was right. Knowing that—even if my breasts don't look like they belong on a model—they do what I ask them to do. I have nursed three babies: each one for 14-plus months. I've never really pumped, and I've always had a plentiful supply of milk. What more is there, really? I wouldn't trade my breasts for anyone else's. They have blessed my children and me."

We survive—and overcome—the pressures of life by learning to love ourselves and our bodies and by entering the changes, fully, and embracing the roles our body parts play, and letting them minister to our families—even as we let go of the girl we were and accept the woman we've become.

THE WEIGHT OF PREGNANCY

Pregnancy is a tumultuous time: nausea combined with uncontrollable cravings combined with a child forming within you. Whether or not you struggled with food before you became pregnant, you will probably find yourself wondering why eating has suddenly gotten so complicated.

Karen had never suffered from a clinical eating disorder, but she was always concerned about her weight. Having just given birth to her fourth child, she was once again trying to lose the baby pounds. "When I became pregnant for the first time, I thought, 'For once I don't have to constantly think about food and weight gain,'" she says. Following the delivery of her eldest boy, she went on fad diets, became active in sports, and lost weight quite easily.

"When I became pregnant with my second, I was on a carb-restricted diet," she recalls. "It was hard for me to see my body becoming larger, but I would say I was more worried about how I would look afterwards."

Nevertheless, following the birth of her middle son, she didn't have time to be concerned about dieting. "I didn't even realize it until someone said to me half a year later, 'Boy, it's sure hard to lose the baby weight, isn't it?' I was disappointed in myself."

Soon afterward, however, she became pregnant again—this time with a daughter. Following the birth, she used Weight Watchers to return to her natural body weight. "I remember after I had lost a lot of the baby weight, someone said to me, 'Once we get to our goal weights, we should go shopping together,' and I thought, 'Do I not look like I'm at my goal weight?'"

So Karen decided to lose even more. "I still worry," she admits. "It almost becomes an obsession. I've actually bought clothes that I know will be too small, just for the motivation to get back into shape!"

It's one thing to be concerned about returning to one's "normal weight." It's another to struggle with an eating disorder while trying to lose the baby weight. And thoughtless comments such as the ones Karen faced can quickly cause a relapse.

Ironically, worry over pregnancy-related weight gain can actually trigger a binge eating disorder or other disordered eating issues.[3]

Women who are anxious about weight gain will often go to extremes, restricting their intake and then bingeing to compensate for the excessive food deprivation due to unrealistic dietary rules. Others foster an "I don't care" attitude and eat mindlessly, feeling that they have lost control of their bodies anyhow and "might as well eat" in the face of inevitable weight gain. Then there are those who fear weight gain to the point of restricting severely, risking harm to the fetus.

Dena had one patient who gained just seven pounds her entire pregnancy because of fear of getting fat. Her eating disorder voice could not overpower the one that told her she needed to eat for her child. Sadly, contrary to popular belief, pregnant women with eating disorders don't automatically have the awakening that they need to eat healthily "for the baby." As a result, what is supposed to be a joy-filled, expectant time is, in fact, filled with despair and fear. No longer are these women risking their lives just for the sake of the eating disorder; they're risking their unborn children.

It's easy to judge this kind of mentality, to say, "I would never starve myself if I had a baby inside of me." But we are inundated daily by society's mantra that "thin is in." Pregnant women are not exempt from these messages. Magazines and tabloids criticize celebrities for weight gain during pregnancy and for lack of weight loss following birth; in many cases, there are photo displays just weeks after a celebrity gives birth showing how quickly some of them got back to their prepregnancy bodies. What they don't often mention is that many, if not most, of these women have personal trainers, private chefs, round-the-clock nannies, and other forms of help. What they also don't acknowledge is that losing weight too quickly after childbirth and going back to the gym too soon is not healthy for any woman, celebrity or not.

Actress Hunter Tylo was actually fired from the series *Melrose Place* because she was pregnant. She was told that her ensuing forty-seven-pound weight gain was a "material change" in her appearance and thus a violation of her contract. The executive producer's position was that because of the actress's pregnancy, she couldn't play what they called a "vixen, seductress and adulteress" with any dramatic credibility.[4] Tylo sued the company and won a settlement for pregnancy discrimination, but the fact remains that there are lingering sections of society that do not accept a woman's bodily changes during pregnancy.

So how do we find the strength to fight society and believe we are beautiful, curves and all?

A HEALTHY MIND-SET

It's hard. Most women don't want to gain weight. Ever. It helps when you know you're growing a human being. But it's still hard. To make matters worse, there's an audience when you're being weighed—the nurses hovering, the doctor measuring your womb, and you, feeling like a distended whale. For those of you who battle disordered eating, this is ten times more difficult. Suddenly you're face-to-face with the fact that you have issues, you're forced to overcome them for the sake of a daughter or son you've never met, and strangers are rating your body on charts and exchanging glances. It's all one big trigger.

Because of this, it's important to know yourself. It's important to know what sets you off so you can avoid these triggers and so you can protect yourself as well as your unborn child. If your trigger is numbers, tell the nurses; say that you need to stand with your back to the screen because otherwise the sight of the numbers might cause a relapse. Explain your disorder to your doctor and ask her to be sensitive when it comes to talking about weight gain. It's important that your ob-gyn know your history with eating disorders so she can help you make healthy nutritional choices while watching for any issues that may crop up. Communication is key, both with yourself and with your health professionals. It's worth braving any potential shame to save a life.

A GENERAL GUIDELINE

A common misconception about pregnancy is the adage "Eat for two." For overeaters, this is often just an excuse to binge even more. Focus instead on eating healthily for one, on eating wholly and completely for yourself. Remember that the baby is not full grown; you're eating for one adult and for an infant who is very, very small. If, however, you've struggled with anorexia in the past, and you find it hard to eat for yourself, then go ahead and eat for your child. *Just eat.* That's what matters. Eat nutritiously and often.

Pregnancy heightens our hunger cues. It allows us to listen to our bodies, to understand whether or not we want protein, calcium, carbs, fruits, or vegetables. Just like learning a baby's cries (hunger, tired, gassy), it takes time to learn the body. Obey your desires—in moderation. Don't use pregnancy as an excuse to overeat, but don't ignore your cravings, either. Be obedient to your body during this time. It knows what it needs (this process is known as intuitive eating and will be discussed further in chapter 7).

PUTTING ON THE POUNDS

Try not to worry about weight gain or calories. Rather, focus on being good to yourself. Allow your pregnancy to be an organic, natural, and beautiful experience during which you fall in love not only with your baby, but also with yourself. This may be difficult to do at first, but if you can be mindful of your body, yourself, and your baby, it may feel easier. You may find that prenatal yoga or meditation helps relax you, dulling the tension that can accompany *having* to gain weight.

That said, the Mayo Clinic does suggest certain habits to help add extra calories nutritiously:

- Trade white bread and pasta for the whole-grain variety.
- Choose a salad with low-fat dressing or black beans instead of a burger and fries.
- Eat sliced fruit instead of a cookie.
- Choose juices fortified with calcium and other nutrients.[5]

When it comes to putting on the pounds, most women should expect to gain about two to four the first trimester, and then three or four each month (or an extra three hundred calories each day) for the last six months (or the second and third trimesters). Divided up, the weight falls into the following categories:

- Baby: 7 to 8 pounds (about 3 to 3.6 kilograms)
- Larger breasts: 2 pounds (about 1 kilogram)
- Larger uterus: 2 pounds (about 1 kilogram)
- Placenta: 1.5 pounds (about 0.7 kilogram)
- Amniotic fluid: 2 pounds (about 1 kilogram)
- Increased blood volume: 3 to 4 pounds (about 1.4 to 1.8 kilograms)
- Increased fluid volume: 3 to 4 pounds (about 1.4 to 1.8 kilograms)
- Fat stores: 6 to 8 pounds (about 2.7 to 3.6 kilograms)

Of course, if you are carrying multiples, the numbers differ. According to the American Pregnancy Association website, "Weight gain depends on a number of factors including height, body type, and prepregnancy weight. However, most women who are carrying twins are encouraged to gain 35 to 45 pounds. Women carrying triplets are advised to gain 50 to 60 pounds."[6] Those carrying more than three are encouraged to talk to their doctor.

While we don't want you to worry about your weight gain, at the same time, it's good to be wise and to know that weight gain is healthy and necessary in pregnancy. If you gain too little, you could harm your child. If you gain too much, you could harm yourself through gestational diabetes, high blood pressure, and preeclampsia. The required amount of weight gain varies by individual and is best discussed with your doctor. Overall, a woman with a healthy prepregnancy weight should generally gain between 25 and 35 pounds, whereas women who are underweight should aim for 28 to 40 pounds. Women with higher body mass indexes might be advised to gain anywhere from 11 to 25 pounds, but it is only in extreme cases that doctors would prescribe medically supervised weight loss of a small amount.[7] If this is all too much to handle on your own, please don't be afraid to ask for help. A nutritionist or dietitian would be more than happy to help you write up menus and talk you through finding your way into health, for the sake of you and your baby.

DOCTOR VISITS

Dena was being weighed at the doctor's office during her fifth month of pregnancy when a nurse declared, "Wow, you have gained seven pounds in one month!" Dena was taken aback by this comment; she felt scolded.

"Could that mean there is something wrong with the baby?" she asked.

"No, most likely you are just pigging out too much," said the nurse.

Dena was later assured by her doctor that there was nothing wrong with the baby. She then admitted to not appreciating what the nurse had said. The comments were very insensitive, she told her doctor; after all, body image disturbances only heighten during pregnancy. The nurse had made her feel she was doing something wrong when in reality, she was eating nutritiously and taking care of herself.

It is easy to fall prey to others' opinions when you're unsure about yourself, when you're bloated and tired and patterned with varicose veins. But in spite of your appearance, your opinion still matters. *You* still matter. And this isn't because you're carrying a human being, although that is certainly a blessing. It's simply because of the fact that you are you.

So carry that worth on your shoulders, stand tall, and stick up for yourself when you're being insulted or discouraged. It doesn't matter whether or not it happens at the doctor's office or on the streets. As the saying goes, "I am woman. Hear me roar!"

Roar gently. Be loving, but don't believe the lies. Don't let the negative opinions of others get you down. And if you're able to be selective, choose your doctor, or your midwife, wisely. Choose someone who will build you up, not tear you down. Because you deserve all the kindness in the world.

NOT A SOLUTION

Elizabeth Stone, author of *A Boy I Once Knew*, said, "Making the decision to have a child—it's momentous. It is to decide forever to have your heart go walking around outside your body."[8]

While pregnancy is motivating and inspiring, it is not a recommended cure for what ails you. As a twenty-two-year-old disordered eater told Dena, "I thought if I become pregnant all my eating disorder issues would go away, because I wouldn't want to hurt my child, but they have just become worse. I hate myself even more now."

Having a baby is *not* the solution to your problems, whether they consist of an eating disorder, marital strife, or loneliness. Nothing can totally prepare you for the journey of pregnancy and motherhood, the roller-coaster of emotions, the changes in relationships and roles, and the exhaustion. So before adding more heads to your home, seek counseling and recovery. Because if you can't take care of yourself now, how are you going to take care of a child?

THE POSITIVE EFFECTS OF PREGNANCY

While pregnancy is not a solution, there is no doubt that it can inspire health and wholeness. The process of producing life allows women to relinquish the pursuit of thinness. It is a time of letting go of dieting, calorie counting, and obsessing about weight gain, all while taking into account another (tiny) person's life. For women constantly on a diet, pregnancy becomes a chance at freedom.

One of Dena's patients, a young mother, told her, "Being pregnant was one of the happiest times of my life, because it allowed me to eat the food I loved . . . interestingly enough, it was healthy food."

Another disordered eater admitted that, during her pregnancy, "I listened to what my body was craving, ate when I was hungry, and stopped when I was full."

Pregnancy is powerful. The love between a mother and child is the only bond stronger than addiction. After all, love is life. And life trumps death. Providing a home for life not only motivates us as mothers, but serves as a token of responsibility to carry this little person to term. Pregnancy thereby motivates us to be better people by acting as a catalyst for change.

The experience also gives us "permission" to see and experience our bodies differently. As priorities change from "What should I eat?" to "How should I live?" inner strength is found, motivating a woman to face—and conquer—her fears on behalf of her child.

YOUR GREATEST ACCOMPLISHMENT

If you struggle with disordered eating or body image issues and are now pregnant, we'd encourage you to embrace this opportunity. Work toward freeing yourself of these destructive behaviors, and walk in wholeness. You are about to enter the most wondrous of communions: creation. You are about to give life. This is art. This is better than any Picasso. And you want it to be gold, to be all that it can be. So eat as though you're worth it.

"Mothers do this thing where we sit around and compare war wounds," writes Lisa-Jo Baker, social media activist and blogger at *The Gypsy Mama*. "We revel in it. Comparing how many hours we were in labor, how the anesthetic wore off, what the doctors said, how large our newborn's head was or how much he or she weighed. . . .

"But in reciting all these lists and comparing all these stories, we are leaving out a crucial element. The only part of the story that really matters . . . the otherworldly experience of co-creating life with Christ. . . .

"It is one thing to picture the Creator shaping Adam from the earth; it is another to feel a human foot kick you from the inside. It is one thing to understand with your head that man was made in his Father God's image; it is quite another to look into the scrunched up eyes of a wailing infant and hear her cries soften as you whisper 'I'm your mama.' . . . It is sacred. It is bloody. It is real."[9]

Giving birth produces life in more than one sense. It's the baby powder, milky-breathed spirit found in the softest limbs you've ever felt, and it's the respect a man feels for his wife as he watches her give up her body for another. And it's the deep-rooted, soul-satisfying feeling of knowing you were born for more than the mirror. That you were born to see the face of God in your child, and to know that you yourself are a miracle.

EMILY'S STORY

We were drinking tea at Auntie Marg's, and I was six months pregnant and bulging with boy. Auntie Marg was beaming, her apple cheeks pink and her white curls, prim. Even though we weren't related, she was family. Margaret and her husband, Uncle Jim, had known me for twenty years. We'd met them when we were living up north, Dad preaching at a tiny church in rural Ontario.

I was married now, and expecting our first son after a miscarriage and a failed adoption attempt. I was listening to my body, eating meat when it wanted meat, and calcium, fruits, carbs, and vegetables, and I carried my womb proudly—like a trophy.

We were drinking tea and Marg was beaming, and we were remembering days of old, when my brother and sisters and I would sleep over in the "loft" and go snowmobiling and listen to Uncle Jim play the fiddle. Then Marg paused and swallowed and said, "You were so thin then. So very thin. I didn't know what to do. And now—" she looked at my arms, "You look so good. So healthy. There is meat on your bones."

It took everything in me not to burst into tears. Instead, I set down the china teacup and searched frantically for Trenton's eyes. And when I found them, I held on like a desperate woman, and he smiled slightly. Even more slightly, he shook his head as though to say, "Don't think it. Don't believe the lies. Because you are beautiful. So very beautiful."

A few years earlier, a comment like Marg's would have sent me spiraling into another eating disorder. The word "healthy" somehow implied I was plump. Not sickly, or skinny, the way I wanted to be. But I was carrying life now. I had learned my body was made for more than turning men's heads. It held the key to regeneration; it was home to a child, and more than that, it was the cord that connected heaven to earth.

My child ate what I ate; if I starved my body, my baby starved. My identity was more than that of a lonely woman, or a little girl desperate for approval, or an artist or a writer or a wife. It was that of a *mother*.

Nevertheless, as Lamott says, we are all the ages we've ever been, and I was a mother stuck in a little girl's head. I was trying, with all my might, to shake off the old way of thinking, but anorexia is a mental illness. Its roots are in the brain, and it takes years to reprogram. Years to reverse the damage that self-abuse has caused.

Auntie Marg hadn't meant to make me cry. But I did, that night, in the confines of our room, against the safety of my husband's chest and our baby in between. I cried for all the damage I'd let those years do, damage that took simple comments and turned them into missiles.

"She doesn't understand—she doesn't know," Trent said into my hair. "She was trying to tell you that she thought you looked good. Don't let it be more than that."

But I still felt fat in my maternity nightgown and belly. Until Trent took my face in his hands and said slowly, so I couldn't miss it, "You are the mother of my child. And you have never been more beautiful to me."

And even though Auntie Marg's comment stung, I realized in that moment that it didn't matter what she'd said or what I'd heard. *Because love had called me perfect.* And the more I believed this, the more I stopped being a disordered thinker. This would be a truth I latched on to, even as I grew bigger and more tired and bloated and then gave painful, thirty-six-hour-birth to the sweetest-faced little boy I could imagine. A truth that would help me handle the shock of my stomach's not immediately deflating after I gave birth. A truth that would sustain me over months of wanting to fit back into my old jeans and struggling to find value in myself in spite of "just" being a body again.

REFLECTION

If you struggle with mental health issues, including an eating disorder, it is important to get help.

The social respect and value of the parental role has been largely diminished in the United States. Institutional support, resources, and funding that might alleviate social and economic burdens associated with parenting are often lacking. Treatment for those struggling with mental issues often focuses on the individual; if it's an adolescent, then it might include the parents. Children, however, are the ones being neglected, both directly and indirectly.

If you are a loved one reading this book in an effort to help, please take this role seriously. The consequences can be devastating and irreversible. It takes courage but someone needs to understand that the love for one's unborn child is sometimes superseded by the addiction, illness, or disorder.

If you are pregnant and struggling with body image, here are some tips for how to enter this new phase of womanhood with courage and grace:

- Accept and embrace your changing body.
- Eat in a way that will sustain a healthy pregnancy (speak with a nutritionist or dietitian; follow prescribed meal plans if given).
- Find accountability partners who can challenge you on your down days and motivate you to care for yourself.
- Pray that your heart, mind, and soul will be healed and readied for the challenges and responsibilities ahead.
- Meditate on scripture and allow yourself to rest, believing that you deserve love just as much as the next person.

TOOLS

For reproductive and pregnancy health, here are some suggested guidelines. The majority of women with eating disorders can give birth to healthy babies if they have normal weight gain throughout pregnancy.

Prior to pregnancy:
1. Achieve and maintain a healthy weight.
2. Avoid restricting, bingeing, and/or purging.
3. Consult your health-care provider for a preconception appointment.
4. Meet with a nutritionist and start a healthy pregnancy meal plan, which should include prenatal vitamins.
5. Seek counseling to address your eating disorder and any underlying concerns.

During pregnancy:
6. Schedule a prenatal visit early in your pregnancy and inform your health-care provider that you have been struggling with an eating disorder. This is very important—as discussed above, if you don't tell your doctor, he or she probably won't ask.
7. Strive for healthy weight gain.

8. Eat well-balanced meals with the necessary nutrients.
9. Find a nutritionist who can assist you with healthy and appropriate eating.
10. Avoid restricting, bingeing, and/or purging.
11. Seek therapy to address your disordered eating, body image concerns, and any underlying issues.[10]

Tips for working with your doctor:

- Be honest—disclose your disordered eating issues, body image disturbances, and/or other mental health issues.
- Stay grounded. Demonstrate confidence and strength in your approach to your doctor by stating your needs and expectations.
- Be assertive with your physician: "This is what I need; these are my concerns."
- Work with a team—a psychologist, therapist, dietitian; appoint a key person to help you with your treatment (typically this is the therapist/psychologist, but it can vary).

CHANGE, ACCEPTANCE, AND MORE CHANGE

Embracing Motherhood

Cleaning and scrubbing can wait for tomorrow,
For babies grow up, I've learned, to my sorrow.
So quiet down, cobwebs; dust, go to sleep.
I'm rocking my baby, and babies don't keep.

—Author Unknown

ONE SMALL STEP FOR BABY, ONE GIANT STEP FOR WOMANKIND

So you spend nine months massaging your womb and purchasing onesies and reading parenting books and attending Lamaze class. Nine months dreaming about how beautiful your child is going to be, how wonderful it will feel to hold him in your arms, and you practice your breathing exercises and tell everyone you're doing a drug-free birth because it's best.

You put earphones to your womb and stream classical music, pack your nail polish and silk nightgown and the poetry book for your husband to read while you're helping your child ease his way into the world. And then your water breaks at three in the morning, and the contractions choke-hold your abdomen. This isn't the way it was supposed to be. Your husband is on the phone with the fire department instead of the hospital because he's half-asleep and you can't find the bag you packed and you're panting and swearing and stumbling around in a soggy stupor. There is no rhyme or reason to your breathing, no "Lamaze," just a desperate attempt to survive your baby's arrival. Soon you're screaming at your husband to drive faster. No poetry or classical music, only the sound of your old life being ripped apart by an eight-pound ball of flesh trying to exit your body as you suddenly realize how small the doorway and how large the intruder.

And then you get to the hospital, and you order the largest dose of drugs you can get, but it's too late, the baby is coming, and there's no time, only you, yelling at the doctor to *pull that baby out*, your face splitting in two as you give birth to the reddest rat you've ever seen. And as you stare at this wrinkly creature, convinced there must be some mistake, you pray to wake up. For it wasn't supposed to be this way. You had plans. You had a checklist. You're not sure where it is, but you had it.

No one warned you. No one told you how unpredictable this meeting your child would be, how unromantic, how messy. And still, after the doctor has stitched you up, and your husband has revived and is handing you belated cups of ice chips, and you're holding your newborn wrapped in soft flannel, you feel nothing. And this isn't right either. You're supposed to feel *something*. Admiration? Adoration? Passionate love? Euphoria? But all you want is for someone to take your child, the one you've been anticipating these past nine months, so you can cry.

It's true that you forget much of the pain in the face of your baby, but you never forget all of it. For some women, labor is beautiful, and even romantic, but for many, it's not. As Nora Ephron says in *Heartburn*, "If pregnancy were a book, they would cut the last two chapters."[1]

With Emily's second pregnancy, the doctor broke her water after nineteen hours of contractions. She was thrust into an intense twenty-four minutes of drug-free pushing and tearing that left her weeping and fetal, unable to do anything but close her eyes for the pain. There was nothing romantic about it. "I realize why women die in childbirth," said Sherry Glaser. "It's preferable."[2]

And for weeks afterward, despite the joy of finally holding her eight-pound, fourteen-ounce Kasher Jude, Emily struggled with feelings of betrayal, anger, and trauma. She felt as though her husband should have been the one to give birth, the one to spare her the greatest pain she had ever known. But he couldn't have. No man can, and this is one of life's greatest curses: man cannot save woman from hell. Yet man is also deprived of knowing the incredible intimacy that carrying and delivering a child produces.

THE SACRED CALLING

In spite of all the pain and the blood, there is a sacredness to giving birth. A miracle that speaks of becoming one with Someone Greater, with the Creator, and a holy hush that descends on the child emerging: with his perfect ears and long eyelashes. There are no words for how it feels to smell your baby's skin and to know he is yours.

"Day's light begins to spread over sky's black," writes blogger Janae Maslowski. "I cry awe at all the women gathered, I whisper thank you to the powerful, tender, and wise hands that usher me in. My feet find the age-old paths trod by all mothers. With hips swaying and murmurs falling off my lips, I surrender and again, again and again.

". . . I vise-grip her hand and stare into green eyes, she counts me through, helping me hold back the holy force. I lunge and breathe, release and flow to partner with my body, this, my opening. . . . I hold the gaze of each in turn—midwife, husband, doula—and I say the words, 'I trust you. I trust you. I trust you. . . .'

"I am told the time is now—push, push, push—three per breath. Baby emerges, they lay the nine-pound body on my chest, we meet skin to skin. I'm all shock and wonder, I stare and mumble. . . . In turn, all of the women hold him, I want him touched and blessed."[3]

Humanity, in all its vulnerability and rawness, is in your arms. You press it close to your breast and your body produces food as easily as it did life. And for a moment, it all makes sense: you being there, you having this body, you needing this love.

GIVING BIRTH TO CHANGE

They don't tell you that you're giving birth to your heart. That labor is more than a few hours in a sterilized environment. That every day of motherhood will rip you open, womb and soul, and that no one will know how to stitch you up. They don't tell you there is no tool to cut the umbilical cord, not really, and that no matter how far the child runs, the cord drags mother behind. They don't tell you that your dreams become your child as you stare into the face of someone so small, so asleep, and see your father's profile in his bones and your husband's lashes on his cheeks, and that you would die a thousand ways so they might live. No, they don't tell you this. And they don't warn you that the first time you let your child down—that you truly, truly let your child down—that you will cry for hours and kneel by his bed and trace the curl of his hair and beg forgiveness, for in giving birth to life, you give birth to death. Death of your former self.

And they don't tell you this as you sob to your husband between the sheets where love conceived life, as you tell him you failed and he promises it's okay and all you can think of is the future and the chance of your son going through worse pain. Then your husband says you must stop, in a stern kind of voice that reminds you that you are not God and you need to stop crying for you are a mother now. And they don't tell you there is a fine line between being mother and being martyr and you cannot be everything for everyone, and the best thing you can do sometimes is fold your hands and pray.

Motherhood has an enormous impact on your relationship with food and body because it affects your mood, feelings, thoughts, and behavior. There is a lot to negotiate. You are *the* one for this child. You will know no one as intimately as you do this little person. You begin to discover changes in your sense of purpose and meaning. Your focus shifts, and priorities change, as your child draws you away from yourself. And while postpartum depression is a very real possibility, sadness can also subside in the face of serving someone else. Babies have a way of taking the heart hostage. Disordered eating, body image concerns, and other issues are often replaced by life. As you answer the call of motherhood, you begin to see who you truly are and what you have to offer.

You're indispensable to this tiny person. And this creates a feeling of worth and security.

BABY BLUES

Pregnancy also results in panic attacks, immobility, and sadness. According to a 2008 article in *Scientific American*, postpartum depression affects one in five women.[4] Brooke Shields suffered a severe case following the birth of her first child. In *Down Came the Rain*, her account of the experience, she writes, "This was sadness of a shockingly different magnitude. It felt as if it would never go away."[5] Fortunately, it did, after Shields reached out for help—an action that saved both her life and her relationship with her baby.

Upon giving birth, every woman will experience, in varying degrees, sadness, confusion, disconnect, loneliness, and fatigue, in addition to an overwhelming sense of awe. Those with anorexia and bulimia have three times the risk rate for postpartum depression as those without eating disorders. Research also shows that postpartum depression in women with diagnosable eating disorders is markedly higher the first three months and tends to remain high the following nine months.

Medical guidance regarding psychiatric medication in general is beyond the scope of this book. However, if you struggle with anxiety, depression, or any other mental illness, we highly recommend contacting your doctor. There is a wide range of medications and treatments available. So don't stay in the dark; love on yourself by getting help.

THE PERFECT MOMMY SYNDROME

In addition to having perfect bodies, society tells us we need to be perfect mommies: jogging six weeks after delivery, owning brand-name diaper bags and strollers and cribs, doing playdates, making organic baby food, potty-training the kids soon after birth, and Baby Einstein-ing them into little prodigies—all while holding down a full-time career.

Okay, that's a bit of an exaggeration, but not by much. Parenting books breed anxiety over a child's natural stages; companies and products make mothers feel inadequate for a job ultimately defined by love.

JoAnn Hallum, a blogger and mother of three boys, puts it this way: "It rained for days. Noses poured, tears flowed, tempers flared and the Mother wished everything would dry up. I cried on the toilet while I told my husband about the laundry that lurked up on me. I was so overwhelmed by messes. My children were naughty. My house was embarrassing. The boys splashed happily in the shower while I cried about socks.

"Everything felt soggy . . . I cried in church too, a little bit. And the preacher said God's will for our life is to follow Him. It's not a destination. It's not retirement, or children leaving home. It's not a clean, sparkling house or a fresh batch of cookies. God's will can be found even in the messy places, because He lives there too. . . .

"Be. Don't just Do. Be the person that follows Jesus in every place, in every circumstance. The overwhelming feeling of failure slowly dripped off, and I picked up a sock and told myself the truth: God cares about people, not footwear and floor polish. When it's raining, and your children are sick and your socks are unmatched and smell like sour earth, be the Mother that shows Jesus' love. Your mission is here. Your mission is now."[6]

It's hard to remember this, though, when the socks remain unmatched and the dishes undone and your baby just fell down the stairs because you forgot to close the gate—again. Those who struggle with disordered eating find all of this particularly hard. Perfectionism propels a mother's relationship with her children, and there is a tendency—especially with anorexics—to be uptight, anxious, and excessively controlling. One of Dena's patients found it difficult to play with her child because she was not getting her chores completed. The compulsion to clean was overwhelming. Another battled with overexercise, to the point where she was spending more time at the gym than with her children, who were two and five.

Anxiety destroys the very bonds that make life worth living. Your children don't need a mother who looks great or does great things. They need a mother who *feels* great. Otherwise they'll think they're constantly disappointing you—a belief that will lead them to self-abusive behaviors, such as eating disorders.

HOW TO BOND AND HEAL

There is nothing perfect, nor dignified, about motherhood—something Emily noted one day while her two-year-old son sat on her back saying, "Ride, horsey, ride!" as she wiped up his pee from the floor. No, there's no dignity. There's only love. Ridiculous, humbling love.

Babies may be small, but they are needy. They cannot do anything for themselves, and they come at the most inopportune time—when we ourselves are in need of rest and healing and comfort. With that in mind, you should realize that it is important to prepare ahead of time for hardship. To know what you are getting into, and to prepare yourself mentally, spiritually, and emotionally for the struggle. When you know your triggers—things that will set off your cycle of dieting, overeating, or worse—it is much easier to make a conscious decision not to fall into the trap. Stress, uncontrollable circumstances, fatigue, depression, and loneliness are all catalysts that may accompany the birth of your child. Hormones are swirling, the baby is colicky, you're not feeling connected, your husband is jealous, and all you want to do is cry and watch soaps.

You know what? It's okay. Allow yourself to grieve. So often we think we have to "have it all together." We don't. Life is tough, but God is good. Make that your mantra, slip into some pajamas, and watch a chick flick. Get to know your baby. Spend hours on the couch together, studying each other's features and sleeping when you are tired and saying no to phone calls until you feel ready. Hire someone to take care of your other children, or let a friend or relative into your home to clean and cook for you. Accept gifts, not visits (if you don't want them). You have earned the right to rest. Don't do anything out of pressure; the first six weeks are yours and your infant's. They're your "baby moon."

After that, you'll feel stronger, braver—possibly slimmer, or closer to your "old self"—and ready to greet the world. But for heaven's sake, give yourself time. And eat a piece of chocolate cake. Or two.

And when you're feeling desperate, hand the baby over to your husband and slip away for some time to yourself, and don't feel guilty about it. Get some fresh air and sunlight. Do some light exercise if you want, or get a pedicure if that's more your style. Take some time to reflect on this new experience, this new person, this new stage of life. Sometimes that's all it takes to realize that what you have is indeed what you wanted all along.

OUR STORIES

Emily

The other morning, I looked at my husband at six thirty and said, "So, I've decided, once again, that I don't want to have any kids." He nodded groggily. "Sounds good." Then we both rolled over and stuffed our faces in our pillows while our children yelled from their beds.

Of course I was kidding. Sort of. Well, it depends on the day. On how many clothes my two-and-a-half-year-old has pulled from the drawers, on how many explosive poops my one-year-old has stained our cloth diapers with (not to mention our surrounding furniture and carpet). On how many gray hairs have sprouted from my thirty-two-year-old scalp.

A friend of mine recently told a story on Facebook that bears repeating. She recounted an incident in which she'd taken off her son's diaper to air out a rash. Then she'd gone to get herself a coffee, and upon her return, had found her little boy pulling poop from his bottom and feeding it to his younger brother.

In spite of such horrors, there are other moments—redemptive moments. Like when my boys hold my face in their chubby hands and trace my features as though marveling that their mother is, in fact, an exquisite masterpiece. When they beg to hold my hand. When they snuggle with me in the mornings; when they say "I lug you" at night.

I am always amazed by how famous I feel in the presence of my children. They never tire of me. Even after we've been with one another all day, they still squeal when they see me. They still run at me full speed and pummel my legs and giggle when I "eat" their bellies. As Erma Bombeck said, "Who else would cry just because you left the room?"

Children are good for the soul and poor for the mind. Not only do mothers communicate in baby babble all day, Backyardigans and Thomas the Train run through their heads as they try to sleep at night. I never used to get headaches. Now, I can count on them show-ing up at least once a day. Or all day. It depends on whether or not the children nap.

But every time I am tempted to complain, I remember that my boys are a miracle. Not just "all children are miracles," but really, truly, because I wasn't supposed to be able to have kids. Doctors told me this when I was thirteen years old, after I nearly died. After I robbed my uterus and my body of anything good. After my younger sisters got their "womanly visitors" while my body remained lonely. At the time, I didn't care. I didn't want kids; I only wanted to get better so I could date boys and go to slumber parties and graduate from high school. A person's sense of foresight is limited by her dreams, and I dreamed only of the next five years.

When my female visitor finally arrived when I was sixteen, I leaped down the halls of my high school because this was amazing in and of itself. But after I got married, children were still not a part of the pic-ture, particularly since I was in the middle of another eating disorder doing another number on my female parts.

Some women are born wanting to be mothers. I was not one of them. I was so afraid of messing up my children—of passing on my "huge" issues to them—and so convinced that the world was a dark and scary place with too many uncontrollable variables, that I decided I was better off not having them. This changed when my sister-in-law, who wasn't supposed to be able to have children—something I'd subcon-sciously taken comfort in—told me she was pregnant. I couldn't even respond. It felt like someone was squeezing my throat. I didn't know I could ache with a baby-shaped sadness. That I could feel the invisible arms of my child before he ever came to be. That I could see his face and kiss his dimpled cheeks and yearn with a spiritual kind of yearning for something I'd never known.

I've never hated myself as I did that night. I hated myself for self-ishly destroying any chance of procreating with my husband, and all so I could be thin. It's funny how being thin can be so important until you realize that it accomplishes nothing except hunger. And for the next year and a half, as we tried to make possible what doctors had said wasn't, we prayed and begged for a miracle.

And in August 2009, God heard our prayers, and it was a glorious eight weeks of talking to our little Papoose and picking out names and buying a bassinette before the blood came. It wasn't the good kind of blood—the kind that would accompany my second pregnancy. No, it was the startling bright stuff that tells you to stop, put your feet up, and prepare for bad news.

After the miscarriage, I smartened up and began to take care of my body as though it was a baby. I dressed in comfortable clothes, gave myself daily vitamins, and fed myself when I was hungry. I loved myself, should God have mercy, again. And this is what having children does. It humbles you. Breaks you. Makes you better than you'd ever thought you could be, and all because of a diapered creature who depends entirely on you.

Sophia Loren, author of *Women and Beauty*, states, "When you are a mother, you are never really alone in your thoughts. A mother always has to think twice, once for herself and once for her child."[7] Motherhood splits you open like a ripe fruit so your children can feed off your virtues.

And when the stick turned pink for the second time, and the ultrasound found a heartbeat, and I was still wondrously nauseous at thirteen weeks, I finally felt like I was doing something right. Don't get me wrong. I was still worried that I would mess up the psyche of my children, but the need to bear life gave me courage. And I knew I wasn't alone. By allowing God to perform within me, I was joining hands with women everywhere—past, present, and future. I was linking with history's umbilical cord that connects centuries and cultures and heartbeats.

And as it says in Genesis, it was good.

DENA

Motherhood: it's not like you can just reach out and grab it for the taking. Just because you push a watermelon through your nostril, so to speak, you are not guaranteed an automatic passage to becoming a mom. No, you gradually, slowly, put on the role, like a pair of shoes. Sometimes it's comfortable—a favorite set of sneakers—but most of the time, it's a pair of high heels leaving you bruised, beaten up, and very unstable.

With so many self-help books out there, I thought I could read my way to motherhood. I mean, my goodness, I was a psychologist whose training was specifically geared toward children and adolescents. I had plenty of opinions on how to raise children, and even taught parenting classes. I owned a dog-eared parenting manual; how could I not be qualified?

I will never forget bringing my brand-new baby girl home for the first time. It was an exhilarating day. It felt like I was playing "house"—you know, the game you played with your girlfriends when you were a child. Except this time, I didn't get to put the baby doll back on the shelf. She was real.

My sister-in-law and her family brought us home in their car. Thirty minutes after they dropped us off and left, I realized that all the baby books given to us by the hospital were still in the trunk of their car. And they lived 660 miles away. I was doomed! I immediately went into hysterics, crying to my husband (who probably thought he was witnessing a scene out of *The Exorcist*) that there was no way I was going to know how to take care of this baby if I didn't have those books. I screamed, "How am I going to know how to feed her and change her diaper if I don't have those books?! Get me those books!" A half hour under my care, and my baby had a poor prognosis with me as a mother. Frantic, my husband drove forty-five miles to meet my relatives and retrieve the necessary literature.

Although retelling this story makes me laugh, it also brings tears to my eyes. I was desperately scared. I didn't know what I'd gotten myself into. Becoming something different is scary because it is unknown. And there are plenty of challenges. Difficulties only Steven Spielberg would know how to capture.

For me, it wasn't postpartum depression I struggled with. It was postpartum *anxiety*. I felt an impending doom, the sense that something terrible was going to happen to my daughter—and that it would be entirely my fault. I worried obsessively. I remember phoning my supervisor at work a few weeks into maternity leave, saying, "I don't know how I am going to come back to work, because I am never going to be able to leave my child ever again." I felt I needed to be with my daughter every second. I even remember being nervous taking a three-minute shower because if I didn't hear my baby, she'd feel neglected.

As irrational as it sounds, the anxiety was real. Eventually, about nine weeks later, I came out of it. I distinctly remember talking to my mother, telling her about my panic attacks and asking, "What is happening to me?"

She remarked, "You are a mother. Your life has changed forever. You will see things differently and feel things deeper." Wise words.

Slowly, things returned somewhat to normal. I began to realize that parenting was not about the ability to control my world and protect my child. Rather, it was about letting go and turning to God.

It actually takes more courage to turn over your fears. Entering motherhood caused me to finally relate to my eating-disorder patients who said they were "afraid of not being afraid." That is, they were afraid of acting brave and then obliviously failing, of letting down their guard and allowing a disastrous consequence. Yet in reality, my hyperawareness couldn't keep my child safe. It just exhausted me.

So I started asking God for help. I started chanting the phrase, "God is in control, I can do all things through Christ who strengthens me. . . . God is in control, I can do all things through Christ who strengthens me." Eventually, I believed what I was saying.

REFLECTION

- How has motherhood lived up to your expectations, and how has it shattered them?
- Do you believe you're doing your best as a mother? Why or why not?
- How do you talk to yourself during the day? Do you use a negative or positive tone?
- How much guilt do you carry around on a daily basis? Are you willing to forgive yourself and unload your burdens?
- What are your motivations for having a child? Are they to cure an ache or to love on someone?

- Are you in a healthy enough place to be able to raise a family? If not, what steps can you take toward becoming whole?

TOOLS

- Connect with other mothers. Do this as soon as possible, for someone is bound to make you feel normal in your abnormal state. It takes a village to raise a child—and a lot of coffee.
- Also, beware of the perfectionistic tendencies that drive you (i.e., rules about the way the household chores are done, or rigidity about your own appearance). If they distance you from your family, they're not worth clinging to. Identify the nature of the need for perfectionism (self-worth, fear, reassurance, etc.). Then repent and allow yourself to make mistakes, one day at a time.
- Have realistic expectations about your body regarding postpartum. It took nine months for the body to change and prepare for birth. It will not revert to its old self overnight. Be patient and kind with your flesh; it's gone through a lot.
- Be mindful of disordered thinking. There is a great deal of societal pressure to lose pregnancy weight "instantly." This unrealistic expectation regarding shape and weight following childbirth can fuel disordered behaviors even in women who did not have these issues previously. Thus, take charge of any negative thinking and self-deprecation. Record over messages that may be playing in your head about how you're "supposed to look" with positive affirmations about who you are and what your body is capable of. Just think: your body created a miracle. That means you're something special.
- Get help for depression, anxiety, or any other psychological issue you may be experiencing.
- Seek spiritual support; talk honestly to God about your fears and frustrations. God is in control, and all things are possible with him. Spend time seeking him, daily, even if it's just minutes in meditation and prayer.
- Communicate. This is *key*. Tell others, and yourself, how you are feeling. Talk, journal, blog, paint, or draw, but use some form of communication.

- Believe in yourself. You are a strong creature made by God. You have been given tremendous abilities. Despite the sleep-deprived nights, the endless days, the foggy brain as the result of being a mother, you are a woman first. And as a woman, you are truly extraordinary, not because of what you do, or how you look, or what you say, but because of who you are. It's that simple!

THE SLEEPLESS WIFE

How to Balance
Marriage and Motherhood

Two imperfect people got married and it was the promise that made the marriage. And when our children were growing up, it wasn't a house that protected them; and it wasn't our love that protected them—it was that promise.

—Thornton Wilder

ON SEX AND SOOTHERS

We're friends, seated around a table talking about our men, and how we love them and need them, but for some reason, they can never seem to get their clothes in the hamper.

Then we get on the topic of lingerie. "It all depends on . . . how much effort I want to put into my marriage," one woman admits.

We nod. We get it. Some days, well, we'd just rather slip into some flannels, read a good book, and fall asleep. And the more we're pulled, prodded, pried, and sucked, all day long, by children with no respect for personal boundaries, the less we desire to be intimate in bed. Not to mention wanting to hide the stretch marks and crow's-feet and Caesarean scars; the flab, where there were once abs, and the boobs, swollen and bruised, or drained and saggy. Because even women who have a healthy body image get these things. They may mind them less, but every woman experiences some change in her body after pregnancy.

But in spite of—or because of—our curves and insecurities, our husbands find us even more irresistible. And we need to honor this. So when do you give in? When do you say, "Honey, I love you, but I love sleep more," and when do you light a candle? Well, it's a given that for the first six weeks (at least) after giving birth, you're off-limits. You've been torn, ripped, and bled dry, and if you've had a C-section, there are the stitches to contend with, not to mention the fragility of your mind. When you've had your female parts exposed to a roomful of doctors and nurses, as well as a child exiting your insides, there's going to be some hesitation about letting anyone near you for some time. After all, making love is what got you into this situation in the first place.

It feels like you'll never need sex again. It feels as though you could happily live in flannels forever, and you consider donating your lingerie to the Salvation Army. But your husband (and your marriage) still has needs, and eventually, your body will recover. The stitches will close up, the flesh will heal, and your pajamas will need to be laundered (and perhaps thrown away).

Because the man who shares your bed is also a priority. Even if it means putting aside your negative feelings about your postbaby body. After all, if your husband is still chasing you around the room, then you can't look that bad!

THE ISLAND OF "ME"

You're in high demand. And all you want is to be left alone. That's why, after the kids go to bed, or during naptime, it's important to vacate to the "Island of Me"—the one between the shores of Motherhood and Marriage, where it's just you, alone with yourself. If you don't, the island (and your personality) will slowly sink, and the two countries will join, leaving no boundaries or borders between the two. Once you've spent even twenty minutes alone on the island, visiting your old hobbies, spending time in quietness, you'll have the strength to switch gears, to cross over to your marriage, having remembered that it is separate from motherhood, and requires your passport as a lover.

When Emily was pregnant with her second son, she felt crowded and overwhelmed: she had the feet of one boy in her ribs and the other crying out to be held while her husband played footsie and touched her flushed skin. All she wanted was to declare "sanctuary"; she longed for a space to call her own. This being a mother, being a wife, is good and blessed, but what do you do when you forget who you are? When the hands beg to be held and the noses wiped and the mouths kissed, and it's no longer just a peripheral thing, for the calling is swallowing up your insides?

And then Emily saw them, walking into church: five children who had just lost their mother. And that's when sanctuary happened. A glimpse into life without the little arms that wrapped her legs or the size 9 feet that played with her toes. She was granted grace to see beyond the spit-up, to see life for what it really was. And this is what she saw: a gift that enfolds us completely.

Finding Ourselves

So how do we find this kind of grace? How do we find the strength to lend our body, to offer our breasts to babe and lover, and to remember, meanwhile, that we are so much more? That our bodies are still ours?

First of all, we need to believe in ourselves. To believe we're not "just" the role we fill, but that we matter, simply because we *are*. We need to hold on to the identity we had before we became this semblance of a person who barely has time to brush her teeth or run a comb through her hair. And then, we need to carve out space and time for ourselves, to honor the soul that lies, fatigued and lonely, beneath our overstretched, overused skin. Because we're more than our flesh, and everyone needs nurturing. And this is no less true when we become mothers.

In fact, we need pampering more often when we spend our days giving to others. But children, as adoring and as loving as they are, are not able to pamper us in the tender way we need. They give, as they can, through kisses and hugs and head pats and smiles, but they take more. And this is the way it's meant to be. We're not meant to lean on our children.

Men sometimes give in a different way, in a "let me fix you" kind of way that rushes over the details and Band-Aids the bruises. Yet it's often the details that mend us, as women: the massages, the soaks in a bathtub, the reading with no distractions. The quiet in which to pray, to reflect, to journal, or to meditate.

Rather than needing someone trying to fix our problems, we need permission just to *be*. The thing is, it's often *we* who need to give ourselves permission.

Born to Break

Even as men tend to fix, women break: they break their backs and hearts in order that the world might be born. But breaking implies that we, too, are at some point whole. So it's a constant reverting to wholeness, letting the fractured places mend so we can break all over again. Labor is, in fact, an everyday breaking for our family. Just as we need to rest between contractions, we also need to rest during the week—to ask our husbands to bathe the kids while we put up our feet; to set aside an hour of personal time each evening, after the kids go to bed.

As women, we need to be kind to ourselves, for we tend to abuse ourselves when life gets too hard. We need to honor our bodies, to know when they need rest, comfort, pampering, and even exercise and nourishment. We also need to honor our souls and our minds, so that we nourish those other parts of our lives that make us who we are.

So take the time to have a bath, to eat nutritiously, to read a book, or to call a friend. When you're grocery shopping, stock up on healthy snacks: granola bars, nuts, fruit, and yogurt for when you can't sit down and eat a full meal. Enjoy a cup of tea in the evenings, or a glass of wine if that's your preference.

Breathe deeply, and laugh at yourself. Laugh at the kids. Laugh with your husband, at the kids. If you feel like you're going to snap, step outside for a minute and stare up at the sky. Slow down, and enjoy the moments of your life that you can steal. Feel your skin and yourself inside of it. Read your Bible, or devotional, or some other form of inspiration either early in the morning, on the toilet, or right before bed. Pop in an educational movie for the children; send your husband out with his buddies, and do something for yourself: paint, or write, or sew. Or ask your husband to stay home while you reconnect with some friends. Check your e-mail. Play your guitar. And don't feel guilty (as long as you do everything in moderation) because the happier you are, the happier your family will be. In short, don't let motherhood or marriage dictate your life. Let there be marriage, motherhood, and ME. This time to yourself will give you the strength to serve: your husband, your children, and your God.

Loving Our Reflections

Lamott calls her thighs her aunties. Perhaps we should find names—kind names—for our ski-slope nose, our pear hips, and wide feet.

With one hand we paint, we write, we strum a guitar; with the other, we change diapers, spoon cereal, soothe foreheads, and sweep up broken goldfish crackers. And sometimes, while our families sleep, we slip to the mirror and pull back our hair and wash our face. We cut our nails and it feels like heaven. We shave our legs and pluck our eyebrows and sing to ourselves as we dare to moisturize. And for a moment, we remember that we are more than mothers. More than wives. We are women. These simple actions remind us of the person who lies beneath piles of laundry and to-do lists and dirty dishes. The woman who dreams. The woman who laughs too loudly and cries too quickly and feels too fiercely. The woman who believes in goodness and trusts too many. The woman who makes her man blush.

Time ticktocks to the rhythm of a child's heartbeat, and when we emerge from the bathroom, we are groomed, pressed, and primed for another day of unraveling, wrinkling, and pulling. And we breathe in the prayer that is our life and remember the face of the woman in the mirror. Because if we forget her, we lose ourselves.

MAKING YOUR MAN MATTER

Once you've called "sanctuary" and put up your feet and remembered who you are apart from the many hats you wear, you need to remember *him*—the man you fell in love with; the man who got you into this beautiful, wonderful, delightful thing called "family" in the first place; the man who says he knows you better than you know yourself, and when you insist, "No you don't," he says he knew you were going to say that.

Upon giving birth, we, as women, have the tendency to mother the romance out of our marriage. Our husband becomes just another task to check off the list. Another voice to appease, another dish to clean, another body to put to bed, another set of hands on our bodies.

"To keep the fire burning brightly there's one easy rule," writes poet Marnie Reed Crowell. "Keep the two logs together, near enough to keep each other warm and far enough apart—about a finger's breadth—for breathing room. Good fire, good marriage, same rule."[1]

The thing is, you've changed: you've carried a living being inside your body for nine months and undergone the excruciating process of labor, and you are now personally responsible for keeping this child alive. On top of that, you still have your daily household duties to fulfill, the scars and the bruises from labor, perhaps a job to do, and other children to care for.

And you're not good with change. You tend to latch on to food when change happens or when stress occurs, and you either don't let yourself eat, or you eat too much, and you don't want anyone touching you or needing you or loving on you because you feel disgusting. And confused. And spent.

And then there's your husband. He hasn't changed—not much, anyway. And he's feeling lonely and useless because, while he can love on this new addition and change her diapers and make her laugh and tell her stories, when it comes to any physical needs such as food, sleep, or comfort, generally only you, the mother, suffice. And for a man who thrives on being needed, whose nickname is often "Mr. Fix-It," this is a huge blow. He wants desperately to help you and your child, but isn't quite sure how.

Delegate

This is where you come in. Instead of trying to take care of everything and everyone on your own, it's important not only to nurture your husband, but to delegate, to spell out ways in which you need him. Suggest the pile of clean clothes that needs folding, or the toys that need picking up; be clear but don't push or force or demand. Men want to help—they just need a gentle nudge. If you have offers of help from others—your mother, your friends, your neighbors —take them up on it. As much as you want to support others in times of need, allow others to help you.

Appreciate

After they've helped you, appreciate them. Do it with respect, not condescension. Pause and look before you talk—see who it is you're addressing, then adjust your voice and words accordingly. Men respond best to admiration. So instead of, "Wow, good job doing the laundry, honey! I'm so proud of you!" say, "Thank you, honey. You're a real life-saver."

Deep down, most men want to be a hero. And this doesn't stop once the kids come along. In fact, it only increases, as they want to be respected by, and in front of, their offspring. In the same way, women—for the most part—want to be cherished and nurtured, to know they are taken care of. Dr. Emerson Eggerichs, author of *Love and Respect*, compares the need for love and respect to that of an air hose. "[A woman] needs love just as she needs air to breathe," he writes. "Picture, if you would, the wife having an air hose that goes to a love tank. When her husband bounds in and starts prancing around like a 10-point buck looking for someplace to graze, he steps on her air hose. This does not make her a happy camper. . . . Simply put, when her deepest need is being stepped on, you can expect her to react negatively. . . . She is not getting the 'air' she needs to breathe. She is crying out, 'I feel unloved by you right now. I can't believe how unloving this feels. I can't believe you're doing this to me.'

". . . The husband needs respect just as he needs air to breathe. He also has an air hose that runs over to a big tank labeled 'respect,' and as long as the 'air' is coming through, he is just fine. . . . Suppose the wife, a lovely doe, starts tromping on his air hose with her sharp little hoofs. [She] may have . . . good reason to prance all over her husband's air hose, but . . . as his air hose starts to leak because of all the little cuts her hoofs have made in it, the husband is also going to react because his deepest need (respect) is not being met. And the battle is on."[2]

Eggerichs refers to this as the "Crazy Cycle."

It wasn't until eight years into her marriage that Emily truly understood the need to respect, as opposed to simply love, her husband. One night Trenton was heading out into the cold to get wood for the stove. He took great pride in heating the house with wood, but Emily didn't feel it was necessary for him to brave the cold that particular night. "Don't worry about it," she said. "We'll just turn on the furnace, and you can stay inside and keep warm." But this made Trenton feel about as old as their toddler. Emily couldn't understand why he'd taken offense to her caring for him, but he didn't want to be treated like one of her children. Instead, he wanted to hear, "Thank you for providing for us. I appreciate you."

This incident marked a turning point in their marriage. The word "appreciate" became a fixed part of Emily's vocabulary, as she realized she couldn't speak to her husband the same way she did to her kids.

Date

In addition to speaking with respect, know your man's love language. Trenton's is "quality time"—a hard one for Emily, who, being an introvert, values her personal space. Taking both of their needs into consideration, each night, after the kids go to bed, Emily and Trent spend an hour alone and then get together to play a board game or watch a sitcom. As Mignon McLaughlin, author of *The Second Neurotic's Notebook*, says, "A successful marriage requires falling in love many times, always with the same person."[3]

It's taken nine years, but in spite of another relapse into anorexia and three years of subsequent insomnia, starvation, and fighting, Emily has nurtured a strong and loving relationship with Trent. It happened in the scalding water, the scrubbing of pan and floor, and the squeezing of breath into nap times. But even more, it happened in the milk of night when Trent would turn as Emily whispered, "I love you," and kiss her hard—only to be interrupted by the raspy cry of a feverish child. She'd go, bending over the crib for fifteen minutes holding her tiny one's fears while her husband waited in the next room. And then she would return to him. Because as wives and mothers, our bodies are often not our own.

The rails of the crib are like the cross: we die to ourselves and hold babies into sleep and then crawl into bed and love husbands into theirs. And afterward, we lie awake, knowing it's all a choice, and we would do it all over again. Because this bending over tired is white-gowned worship, a holy way of being woman.

REFLECTION

- Do you carve out time each day for yourself, or do you spend every minute serving others?
- How often do you take the time to remember who you used to be, before you got married or had kids?
- Do you find yourself resenting your husband for wanting to spend time with you?
- How often do you treat yourself to a pedicure or some other indulgence to make you feel better about your body?
- Do you delegate, appreciate, and date your husband?

TOOLS

- Make an effort to spend at least fifteen minutes a day treating yourself: indulge in a face mask, a book, a nap.
- Plan a date for you and your husband, one that honors the people you were when you first met.
- Practice noticing the little things your husband does around the home, and thanking him.

BEYOND BREAST MILK (OR FORMULA)

The Challenges of Feeding Children

*No one could give her such soothing and sensible consolation
as this little three-month-old creature when he lay at her
breast and she felt the movement of his lips and the snuf-
fling of his tiny nose.*

—Leo Tolstoy

FEEDING FRENZY

It started off easy. You fed them milk or formula. End of story.

Well, maybe it wasn't easy—maybe it was sore and tiring and made you feel like a cow—but there were just two choices: breast milk or formula, and you didn't have to worry about calories or nutrients or whether or not your babies were full because they came with everything necessary to gauge their internal diet.

Then they hit six months, and it came time for cereal. And you started to panic. There are all kinds of cereals, and you're choosing whether to mix it with water or breast milk or formula and suddenly your child doesn't want to nurse anymore, he just wants solids. So you mash carrots and strawberries and potatoes and he spits them out and you begin to feel anxious. Because food makes you anxious. For many people, it's an easy, beautiful thing, but for you, food is hard. Perhaps you need it too much, as evidenced by the chip crumbs in your bed sheets. Maybe it satisfies a void larger than your stomach, and you can't find enough cookies to fill that empty, aching space. Or maybe you're so afraid of needing it that you don't let yourself eat at all. Whatever the case, you do not have a normal relationship with food. And suddenly, your baby is looking at you, needing you to teach him how to eat. And you want to throw in the towel (and the bib) and call it quits.

Take a moment and breathe. Step away from the counter, relax your hold on the spoon, and see your child for who he is: a second chance. A chance to learn to love yourself again. To learn to love food again. And to learn to love God.

IT'S NOT ABOUT FOOD

It was never about food. Food is a means for staying alive; taste buds are a perk. They allow food to be enjoyed, but the actual act of eating is very mechanical and natural. It serves as gasoline for the car. So it's not about the food.

No, it's about *you*. When you believe that you are damaged, that you are not as good as the next person and will never measure up, then all your decisions, all your thoughts and hopes and dreams and everything that you say are a source of shame. You feel you need to hide yourself, like Adam and Eve in the garden when God came looking for them. And there are no fig leaves big enough.

It's hard for you to choose anything because you can't trust yourself, and life is one big menu, full of choices, and the server (your family, your friends) is standing there waiting for you to mess up. A diet is a way to assert control, to both punish and feel good about yourself. You are unsure about everything, so you choose to focus on one thing, food, because it is tangible. You can measure it and control it, or abuse it and yourself by eating too much, and no one can stop you. It's the one thing you have, and you're holding fast. Until you realize that food isn't even beginning to touch the places that ache to be filled and you're left lonelier and emptier than ever before.

Your existence is not something to apologize for. You are a beautiful, intentional creation who was designed for a specific purpose on earth. And until you stop feeling ashamed and start claiming forgiveness and walking in grace, you will never discover your true identity. This walking, this claiming forgiveness, doesn't come easily. It's a retraining of the mind and soul. But it doesn't matter if you feel it. Just work on knowing it. Know you are worth getting up for, and putting on makeup for, and eating nutritiously for, and laughing for. Know there is a divine artist who painted you with such tender brushstrokes he would die to save you. And he did: he died to save you. Because you are his masterpiece. You are loved. And the more you walk in this knowledge, the more the feelings will follow.

Since the beginning of time, since Eve said no to God and yes to temptation, she also said yes to the lie that God no longer loved her. The lie that, if he did love her, he would have said she could eat from the tree. Whether or not you take stock in the biblical story of creation, there is no doubt that females struggle to believe they are valuable. We don't think we deserve to be loved. We don't think we deserve gifts, like food. Yet, in the same breath, we believe that our children—who are unable to earn love—are more than deserving of it. Why is this? When does a child or person stop being deserving? And when, if ever, will we learn to treat ourselves with kindness?

"It's hard to find a photo with the kids that has me in it," writes Baker at *The Gypsy Mama*. "When did I stop considering myself photoworthy? Because, after all, when I hunt for beauty, it is waiting everywhere for me. That nearly six-year-old boy that swoons when I get up in the morning . . . 'Mama, you are so beoootiful!'

". . . Beauty is hiding in the bathroom when I get down on hands and knees to clean the floor and locked in the hot, hot car when I open doors and drive every day to pick up kids with smiles and plans for the afternoon.

"Beauty lingers all around me at two a.m. when I'm up with my baby girl. . . . The more haggard I feel in the morning, the more beautiful I know my soul is becoming.

"This aching for service, for this family. This fighting down frustration and fighting back chaos. This making time in the midst to sit out on the messy back deck with Peter to just reconnect. This is the greatest finding of beauty in the midst of my every-day Polaroid's. My mirror is no longer the boss of me. I now tell it what to see."[1]

DISORDERED FEEDING, DISORDERED EATERS

Feeding your baby—a critical task of early parenting—is a form of communication between you and your child. It allows for your little one to explore the various states of hunger and satiety, and to experiment with autonomy, coordination, and a variety of foods. This aspect of parenting can be overwhelming for mothers who struggle to feed themselves. And if they have a child who has difficulty eating, it can be even more stressful. The challenge begins with breast-feeding. Studies show that "latching and weaning" children may be compromised by women with a disorder. Some women actually use this form of feeding as a way to purge, by not receiving enough calories to sustain their nutritional output, thus losing weight.

When it comes to solid food, disordered eaters also tend to hurt their children due to warped perceptions of portion size and nutrition. Because of the nature of the struggle with eating (control of food, counting calories, fear of weight gain) women with anorexia nervosa may restrict their children's food intake, while those with bulimia nervosa or binge eating disorders inadvertently impose fears of overeating on their children.

"Chronic dieters and health food fanatics can instill food fears, as well," says Ann Capper, RD, CDN, nutrition adviser and editor at FINDINGbalance, a nonprofit organization dedicated to helping individuals eat well and live free. "Then there are emotional eaters, who can train children to soothe with food, while stress eaters can teach them to medicate with food. Such food-centered mindsets can lay the groundwork for children developing full-blown eating disorders when they get older." Despite being born with an innate knowledge of how much they need and when they need it, these children get confused and begin to distrust their own natural instincts.

Dena facilitates an eating disorders group for mothers in which they discuss issues related to parenting. Most often, feeding is the topic of conversation. Common laments include: "I get anxious about over-feeding my children," "I get overwhelmed with cooking," "I am stressed about shopping for food."

One mother shared that she would often get impatient with her son when he was trying to feed himself because "he makes a mess and takes so much time." She said that she couldn't help her frustration. She would constantly be wiping him clean and intruding on his attempts to feed himself. This mother was extremely anxious. Feeding was a chore for her, and without realizing it, she made it a chore for her son.

Another mother said that in the process of preparing meals for her three-year-old daughter and one-year-old son, she would graze off the leftover food from her son's high chair. This would put her in a frenzy, and due to her own guilt, she'd feel frustrated at her son for not finishing his food. She also admitted to giving her daughter less food than her son, even though her daughter was older, for fear her daughter would gain weight. This is not uncommon for mothers with disordered eating or full-blown eating disorders.

For such mothers, instead of being a tool for uniting the family, food becomes divisive—something that is "right" or "wrong"—and mothers become immobilized by calories and content, letting their low self-esteem rule mealtimes. Food itself turns into a weapon or a reward, a way of punishing or bribing children; as a result, extremes occur. Some women withhold fast food and sweets; others deny any structure or boundaries for fear their child will develop an eating disorder. The emotions of those struggling and trying to recover from an eating disorder run the gamut.

Eva, a mother recovering from anorexia, shared that, as a child, she loved Slim Jims, and remembered taking them in her lunch to school. Her own daughter, who is eight years old, discovered Slim Jims through a friend and asked her mother to buy them for her. When Eva looked at the fat content, she was shocked. "I couldn't do it!" she told Dena. "I could not buy this for my child. It was loaded with fat. I do not want my child to be fat." Eva's black-and-white thinking, as well as her anxiety about food, body image struggles, and fear of weight gain, was depriving her daughter of the joy of eating. It was also prohibiting Eva's ability to feed her child "normally," and causing friction among family members, as no one was allowed to eat anything beyond what Eva deemed "safe foods."

Do you eat with your family? Do you share meals with your children? Many mothers with whom Dena has worked don't even sit with their families during mealtime, let alone eat the same food. As one mother put it, "There is a disconnect." This same mother described how her seven-year-old daughter asked her, one evening, why she wasn't eating french fries like the rest of the family.

"Mommy doesn't want to get fat," she told her daughter.

The daughter responded, "Mommy, am *I* fat because I eat french fries?"

Unable to trust themselves when it comes to eating, mothers with eating disorders impose this distrust on their offspring, thereby (unintentionally) raising a generation of fearful children—girls and boys who learn to associate food with anxiety, and subsequently turn into dieters, bingers, and anorexics.

"To treat eating disorders in America is to treat our culture," writes Mary Pipher. "We need a revolution in our values and behavior. We need to define attractiveness with much broader parameters, so that most women, not an infinitesimal few, can feel good about their appearance. . . . Prevention, rather than treatment, needs to be our primary goal. If we can change the way we raise our children, the way our media portrays women, and the attitude we have toward our bodies . . . our daughters (and sons) will grow up strong, healthy, and proud."[2]

INTUITIVE EATING

Before we can feed love—and food—to our children, we need to learn to feed ourselves. To look in the mirror and tell it what to see. To declare ourselves beautiful in spite of our physical reflection. To allow ourselves to believe that we deserve goodness, simply because we exist. True love is taking the time to care for ourselves without compromising the needs of others. As Baker told Emily one day, "That's why I eat brownies, sometimes, for breakfast."

Once we believe we are worth eating for, we can learn to eat intuitively. According to Evelyn Tribole, MS, RD, and Elyse Resch, MS,

RD, FADA, founders and authors of *Intuitive Eating: A Revolutionary Program That Works*, the process consists of ten steps, or beliefs.

1. **Reject the Diet Mentality.** Throw out the diet books and magazine articles that offer you false hope of losing weight quickly, easily, and permanently. Get angry at the lies that have led you to feel as if you were a failure every time a new diet stopped working and you gained back all of the weight. If you allow even one small hope to linger that a new and better diet might be lurking around the corner, it will prevent you from being free to rediscover Intuitive Eating.

2. **Honor Your Hunger.** Keep your body biologically fed with adequate energy and carbohydrates. Otherwise you can trigger a primal drive to overeat. Once you reach the moment of excessive hunger, all intentions of moderate, conscious eating are fleeting and irrelevant. Learning to honor this first biological signal sets the stage for rebuilding trust with yourself and food.

3. **Make Peace with Food.** Call a truce, stop the food fight! Give yourself unconditional permission to eat. If you tell yourself that you can't or shouldn't have a particular food, it can lead to intense feelings of deprivation that build into uncontrollable cravings and, often, bingeing. When you finally "give-in" to your forbidden food, eating will be experienced with such intensity, it usually results in Last Supper overeating, and overwhelming guilt.

4. **Challenge the Food Police.** Scream a loud "NO" to thoughts in your head that declare you're "good" for eating under 1,000 calories or "bad" because you ate a piece of chocolate cake. The Food Police monitor the unreasonable rules that dieting has created. The police station is housed deep in your psyche, and its loudspeaker shouts negative barbs, hopeless phrases, and guilt-provoking indictments. Chasing the Food Police away is a critical step in returning to Intuitive Eating.

5. **Respect Your Fullness.** Listen for the body signals that tell you that you are no longer hungry. Observe the signs that show that you're comfortably full. Pause in the middle of a meal or food

and ask yourself how the food tastes, and what is your current fullness level?

6. **Discover the Satisfaction Factor.** The Japanese have the wisdom to promote pleasure as one of their goals of healthy living. In our fury to be thin and healthy, we often overlook one of the most basic gifts of existence—the pleasure and satisfaction that can be found in the eating experience. When you eat what you really want, in an environment that is inviting and conducive, the pleasure you derive will be a powerful force in helping you feel satisfied and content. By providing this experience for yourself, you will find that it takes much less food to decide you've had "enough."

7. **Honor Your Feelings without Using Food**. Find ways to comfort, nurture, distract, and resolve your issues without using food. Anxiety, loneliness, boredom, and anger are emotions we all experience throughout life. Each has its own trigger, and each has its own appeasement. Food won't fix any of these feelings. It may comfort for the short term, distract from the pain, or even numb you into a food hangover. But food won't solve the problem. If anything, eating for an emotional hunger will only make you feel worse in the long run. You'll ultimately have to deal with the source of the emotion, as well as the discomfort of overeating.

8. **Respect Your Body**. Accept your genetic blueprint. Just as a person with a shoe size of eight would not expect to realistically squeeze into a size six, it is equally as futile (and uncomfortable) to have the same expectation with body size. But mostly, respect your body, so you can feel better about who you are. It's hard to reject the diet mentality if you are unrealistic and overly critical about your body shape.

9. **Exercise—Feel the Difference**. Forget militant exercise. Just get active and feel the difference. Shift your focus to how it feels to move your body, rather than the calorie-burning effect of exercise. If you focus on how you feel from working out, such as energized, it can make the difference between rolling out of bed for a brisk morning walk or hitting the snooze alarm. If when you wake up, your only goal is to lose weight, it's usually not a motivating factor in that moment of time.

10. **Honor Your Health—Gentle Nutrition**. Make food choices that honor your health and taste buds while making you feel well. Remember that you don't have to eat a perfect diet to be healthy. You will not suddenly get a nutrient deficiency or gain weight from one snack, one meal, or one day of eating. It's what you eat consistently over time that matters; progress, not perfection, is what counts (reprinted with permission).[3]

ON TRUSTING OUR CHILDREN

After learning to eat intuitively, we need to learn to trust our children to do the same, to believe them when they say they're hungry or full, and (unless they are obviously over- or underweight), to make nothing more of food than this: an opportunity to sit down with them and connect. Every meal is a chance to commune together, to say grace to a God who has given us this daily bread. By talking, laughing, and relating over plates full of steaming food, children will learn to associate mealtimes with love.

Additional ways to encourage health within our families, according to Pipher, include:

1. De-emphasize the importance of physical appearance in how you describe or evaluate yourself, your children, and others.
2. Don't turn eating and weight into moral issues. Do not use food as a reward or a punishment.
3. Insist that your children exercise at least five minutes a day. The best way to get them started is to set a good example.
4. Give your children the gift of your time, instead of sweets.
5. Don't put your children on diets. Do buy and serve healthy foods, and teach them about healthy eating habits.
6. Have family meals several nights a week. Everyone can help prepare the meal, which should be simple and nutritious. During these meals, turn off the television and do not answer the phone.
7. Plan family fun that isn't connected to eating. Most children love the outdoors and events that involve exercise, such as family roller blading or hikes.

8. Limit your child's television viewing. TV promotes sedentary lifestyles, lookism, and weightism.
9. Limit your children's exposure to magazines and other media that suggest that appearance is a person's most important quality. Discuss with your children media's stereotypes about the obese and the beautiful.
10. Teach your children consumer skills, including a healthy skepticism about advertising.[4]

More than teaching your children how to eat, you are saying that it is *okay* to eat. That it is good to eat. That food is a gift, and they are worthy of this gift, and you are, too. When you begin to worry about whether or not your children have had enough vegetables that day, and whether or not they've eaten too many carbs and not enough protein, remember that food is not as complicated as it seems. And that sometimes, you just have to try.

"Slowly I have realized that I do not have to be qualified to do what I am asked to do," writes Madeleine L'Engle, "that I just have to go ahead and do it, even if I can't do it as well as I think it ought to be done. This is one of the most liberating lessons of my life."[5]

OUR STORIES

Emily

Aiden is at the table, bib around his neck and a sandwich in his hand, and I feel good about what he's eating. It's whole wheat and protein and he has a yogurt and milk. I'm eating well, too—cheese and lettuce on bread—but I can't stop staring at the back of his two-year-old neck in his collared church shirt.

And then it hits me. We're both eating alone: me by the counter and him in his booster seat. I've taken to multitasking lately: to returning phone calls while my sons play with Play-Doh, to putting the dishes away while eating toast while feeding cereal to my youngest son while Aiden sits alone in his booster, but I am struck today by the length of his neck shooting up from his shirt. There will always be more dishes. There won't always be a child in the booster seat.

And this, what it means to feed your son: to sit beside him, as I do then; to look him in the eyes while I take a bite of sandwich and to place a hand on his. To watch crumbs spill from his mouth splitting wide in a smile. I am learning to travel slowly. To taste, to delight. Because life is in the details. In making the most of everything.

Just the other day I was working on a manuscript, absentmindedly eating a bowl of Cheerios, when Trent asked if I had put strawberries in my cereal.

"No, I don't have time for strawberries," I said.

I heard a knife chopping, and soon Trent was standing over me, sliding red berries into my bowl.

"There's always time for strawberries," he said.

I grew up in a house that viewed food as a necessity. We salvaged it, moldy; we reused tea bags until they fell apart in the water; we drank skim milk because it was cheap; and if we didn't finish our plates, at the end of the week we ate Saturday Stew—a conglomeration of the week's leftovers, whether they be spaghetti or meatloaf or liver and onions. We didn't have much money, and we didn't believe in lavishing the money we *did* have on something that only exited our bodies. Occasionally we were treated to day-old doughnuts, and Mum—a nutritionist—would make a delicious zucchini chocolate cake; she also cooked unique meals depending on the country we were studying in homeschool, so we developed diverse palates. But overall, food was merely a "side dish," versus something to get excited about.

Trenton's family was also poor, but the money they made as farmers was put largely toward food because they grew food, and every mealtime honored the work of their hands. If one of her children didn't like the dish she had cooked, Trent's mother made another; she never wanted to fight at the dinner table.

We don't condone either family's method, except to say they're both right and they're both wrong. Balance is best. Food is just food, but it's also an incredible gift. This is why Trent believes in putting strawberries in cereal, why he panics when my toast sits for five minutes ("It's getting cold, Emily!"), and why he says things like, "I put a lot of feeling into those eggs" when he makes an omelet. For Trent, food is a love letter. He doesn't stress about nutrition or weight; rather, he is much like a child when it comes to eating. He eats when he's hungry, he eats in moderation, and he stops when he's full.

I am learning to trust my children, to not worry about portion size or health and to view food as a way to communicate love. But I haven't always done this. In the beginning, when Aiden turned six months and started on solids, I panicked. I studied voraciously, books like *Home Cooking for a Healthy Baby and Toddler* by Martha and David Kimmel and *Wholesome Meals for Babies and Toddlers* by Paragon Books, but I quickly burned out trying to make the perfect meal and watching him spit it all out, mouthful after mouthful.

"Just keep it simple," Trent would tell me.

I didn't want to mess up my child. I wanted to give him the best. Little did I realize that in spite of cooking minestrone soup, and chicken and pineapple cheese, the anxiety I felt was doing more damage than the food was doing good. So I scaled back. I still served nutritious food, but I focused more on the attitude I was feeding with rather than the bowl I was feeding from.

Something I've learned is that in spite of my healing, I still can't trust myself completely. Portion size remains very confusing for me; I tend to cook too much, and serve too much, for fear of my children going hungry. This distorted perception applies not only to food, but also to concepts such as money and material goods. I have learned to rely on the people God has put in my life, to ask Trent how many potatoes to cook, or how much money to spend. It's humiliating that anorexia has affected my life in this way, but it's good to be humbled, to depend on those who love you.

In many ways, I am glad I have boys. I worry that I would mess up a girl. She might see me worrying and think she needs to worry too: about life, about God not being as good as she hoped he was, about boys and school and everything in life that weighs a person down. And I worry these fears would make her try to hurt herself, for her not being able to save the world. Yet boys are people too, and they too have feelings and hearts, and what it comes down to is this: I need to stop worrying so I don't mess up my children. I need to learn to trust God more and take myself more lightly. I need to learn to laugh at myself. In many ways, I need to think less of myself, and a whole lot more about

God. Less of me. More of him. Less of me. More of him. And one of these days, I'll stop worrying about how much I worry, and I'll learn to just live.

Dena

I was chatting with my best friend, who is also a psychologist with two children, and we were grumbling about cooking. To my surprise, my colleague shared a similar dread of grocery shopping, meal planning, and food preparation. It is anxiety provoking, exhausting, and just plain difficult. I think more women feel like this than not. I confess: I do not like to cook. I get overwhelmed trying to make meals for my children. I used to worry about feeding them healthy and balanced meals; this provoked my anxiety and hence my negativity toward cooking. It didn't help that my children were finicky eaters. It was agonizing getting a meal on the table that they wouldn't balk at, loudly.

Do you feel this way? Do you experience a whirlwind of emotions around grocery shopping and food in general? Do you want to do the right thing, but feel paralyzed by choices?

While I've learned, over the years, that food is a lot less complicated than it seems, sometimes I still have trouble organizing dinner. As a result, my kids will often get a piece meal: "Here are your vegetables, son," and then five minutes later, "Oh, and here are your mashed potatoes; the meat will be done in about ten minutes." I laugh with them and say, 'Only in a restaurant will all your food come out at the same time.'" But I have learned to manage and do the best I can. And in the process, I've learned that food is more than it appears.

REFLECTION

- What keeps you from trusting your body completely?
- What keeps you from trusting your children to know what they need to eat?
- Do you force/entice your child to finish the baby food jar or clean his plate, even when he shows signs of being full?

- Do you give your child a cookie any time he is hurt or upset in an effort to comfort him?
- Do you routinely use food to bribe or reward your children?
- Do you gobble up leftovers from your children's plates for fear of waste (discarded pizza crusts, cold potatoes, soggy crackers), thereby treating your body as a garbage can and not as the temple that it is?
- Are you more afraid of getting cancer or of becoming fat?
- Does feeding your children, and yourself, make you anxious? Why or why not? Do you view food as nourishing fuel to be enjoyed?

TOOLS

- **Inspire a positive relationship with food**. Our goals in feeding our children should be to help our children rely on internal cues of hunger and fullness. The guideline provided to us by the Academy of Nutrition and Dietetics is that we eat with "balance, variety and moderation."[6]
- **Trust your children**. Ellyn Satter, RD, an internationally recognized authority on eating and feeding, wrote *Child of Mine: Feeding with Love and Good Sense*. In it, she states: "You are responsible for the *what*, *when*, and *where* of *feeding*. Your child is responsible for the *how much* and *whether* of eating."[7]
- **Create "to-do" lists**. Make lists that help you plan meals, shop, and cook. Sandi Richard's cookbooks come with preplanned grocery lists and nutritious meals that will ease your burdens significantly.[8]
- **Delegate**. Enlist your husband or partner to do the shopping or cooking.
- **Have realistic expectations**. Goals like "I must make a home-cooked balanced meal for my children every night" only set you up for failure. Be kind to yourself.
- **Eat together as family**. It's essential to eat one meal together every day. A study of family eating patterns, published in 2005 by the National Center on Addiction and Substance Abuse (CASA)

at Columbia University, found that family dinners get better with practice; the less a family eats together, the less healthy the food and the more meager the talk. Among those who eat together three times a week or less, 45 percent say the TV is on during meals (as opposed to 37 percent of all households), and nearly one-third say there isn't much conversation. Kids from such families are also more than twice as likely as those with frequent family meals to say there is a great deal of tension among family members, and they are much less likely to think their parents are proud of them.

- **Seek professional help**. It's important to seek help when it comes to discerning between the "eating disorder" voice and the "healthy you" voice. Because it all gets muddled sometimes, you need someone to keep you accountable and sane.
- **Reframe food**. Keep food in the kitchen; put it in its place.

FOOD FROM HEAVEN

Spiritual Nourishment for You and Your Family

*Dear God . . . help the mother . . . help all mothers ev-
erywhere. We need so much help, with the little, sensitive,
loving hearts and minds that look to us for guidance and
love and understanding.*

—L. M. Montgomery, *Anne of Ingleside*

A HUMBLE CALLING

More than healthy eating, more than loving ourselves, is learning to
listen for the still, small voice that tells us the love and wisdom
we need to hear. Once we learn to listen to this voice, we won't be so dependent on the other one: the louder, more abrasive voice that focuses
on our looks, or our talents, or our achievements. It's the still, small
voice that speaks of our eternal value. Of the fact that we were made to
serve and to care for each other, that we matter simply because we *are*.

But to hear the truth about our identity—that we were born for
a higher purpose—requires the utmost humility. Because if you think
you have all the answers, you'll never hear anything. Humility does

not consist of thinking poorly about ourselves. Rather, it is the art of putting ourselves aside so we might make way for something greater, something the whole world is longing for: a deeper kind of meaning. This humility, this realizing our ribs are formed from dust—and will one day return to dust—is all we can hope to teach our children. That while we are lovable, and worth eating for, we are also significant only because we were designed by a Heavenly Father.

"I'm no pilgrim at Tinker Creek, no recluse at Walden Pond," writes Ann Voskamp, author of the *New York Times* bestseller *One Thousand Gifts*. "I live with the broken bodies. . . . The world I live in is loud and blurring and toilets plug and I get speeding tickets and the dog gets sick all over the back step and I forget everything and these six kids lean hard into me all day, to teach and raise and lead, and I fail hard and there are real souls that are at stake and how long do I really have to figure out how to live full of grace, full of joy—before these six beautiful children fly the coop and my mothering days fold up quiet? How do you open the eyes to see how to take the daily, domestic, work-day vortex and invert it into the dome of an everyday cathedral? Could I go back to my life and pray with eyes wide open?"[1]

This praying with eyes wide open, this being real and vulnerable and humble before your children, while reaching up toward heaven, is perhaps the most powerful lesson you can give your family—to teach them that it takes faith to move mountains, and faith to make mothers. The most powerful way to learn, and teach, this humility is to say sorry to your children. It is to apologize when you, as a parent, do wrong by them. It is agonizing and brutal and extremely redemptive, and it gives a child the opportunity to practice forgiveness.

These practices of repentance and forgiveness are necessary. We forget that relationships require more than physical care. We need to take care of each other's hearts. We all have souls, and we all have destinies, and we need to be respectful of these—even the young ones. And one way in which a parent can respect her child is by acknowledging when she has been hurtful or wrong. A parent who admits to being wrong is no less of a person. Rather, this admission shows that she is capable not only of admitting fault, but also of desiring to do, and be, better.

This apology is all Emily ever wanted. For her parents to come into her bedroom and say, "We're sorry for your pain. We're sorry we don't understand. We're sorry that this is happening to you, and will you forgive us?" Emily did eventually hear these words—ten years after recovering from anorexia. Her parents flew out to her home when she was newly married, and they held hands and prayed together. It was perhaps one of the most spiritual experiences of her life. As children, we know our parents are human. It's just nice when they acknowledge it, too. And this is something we can take comfort from daily. In spite of our imperfections, God is bigger. His love is incandescent and omnipotent and he redeems our poorest, and our best, efforts, over and over again.

LEARNING TO LET GO

Trent and Emily were sitting at the dinner table, their son's food untouched and him asking "down," and they hadn't read the Bible yet. But no amount of forcing their boy to sit on a hard wooden chair was going to make him eat or believe, so they let him down. They let him down to play while they read the story anyway, the story about the prodigal son, and all they could hope was that the beauty reached him where he was playing on the floor—the beauty of a God who desperately loves, who runs down the driveway to meet a son who insulted him, who dies for a world that mocks him, who abandons the ninety-nine sheep for the one, and none of it makes any sense. Because it's grace.

And so, we try to parent in a way that doesn't make sense. We try to choose gentleness when anger would be easier. We try to hug our children a thousand times a day and to tell them that they're special even after they've spilled juice all over the kitchen floor, and we keep applauding, keep apologizing, keep adoring, even though they refuse to put their bath toys away and scream when we tell them no.

Because it's grace, in the end, that prays over our children when we can't find the words. It's grace that speaks to the boy on the floor playing with toys. It's grace that will find our children on their deathbed and convince them of truth as they're longing for heaven. And it's grace that helps us breathe when we're afraid we will break, for the heaviness of it all. For needing our children to believe, more than anything else on earth.

WHY SPIRITUALITY MATTERS

When you feed your soul, you feed your sense of self-worth. And this, in turn, shapes your body image. The more you realize your spiritual worth, the less dependent you feel on your body to define you. And this sets you, and your children, free to focus on eternal values and purpose, versus the temporary.

According to the Mental Health Foundation, spirituality is comprised of the following:

- A sense of purpose
- A sense of "connectedness"—to self, others, nature, "God," or Other
- A quest for wholeness
- A search for hope or harmony
- A belief in a higher being or beings
- Some level of transcendence, or the sense that there is more to life than the material or practical
- Those activities that give meaning and value to people's lives.[2]

Feeding your soul is as important as feeding your body. If we don't tend to our souls, we neglect who we truly are and become dependent on the superficial: aspects of ourselves that will fade with time. The soul never fades. It is the eyeglass through which we view life; it defines the parameters of our relationships with others and ourselves. It is art and song and dance, it is poetry, and it is love. And how do we feed it? By allowing light, not darkness, into our bodies. By listening to uplifting music and reading encouraging books and surrounding ourselves with inspiring people, by focusing our thoughts on God at the beginning and at the close of each day, and by refusing to let stress or worry or anxiety cloud our minds and our hearts.

Feeding our souls, in turn, feeds our sense of worth and purpose. After all:

- Faith in God implies that you were dreamed of by a Divine Being before you were born, and that a heavenly home exists for you after you die, providing affirmation and motivation beyond anything the world has to offer.
- Faith in God offers hope and strength. It is divine. There occurs a transformation in which the lies of the past are replaced by God's Truth.
- Spiritual nourishment is essential to seeing yourself as whole. As you allow yourself to be filled with love and grace, you'll begin to see with new eyes. Others will also begin to see you in a new light. Beauty is reflected from the inside out.
- Spiritual nourishment also gives one's family a sense of identity; it provides a platform for values, traditions, celebrations, and practices. In times of struggle, a family's faith may be the substance that provides stability and security.

WHAT SPIRITUAL NOURISHMENT LOOKS LIKE

We who struggle with eating and hardship and hurt tend to be beauty seekers. We run after the aesthetic, desperately desiring a beautiful family and home. But beauty is more than a Maybelline kind of look. It's about laughter lines and curves and angles and shapes; it's about fitting in and glowing and being effervescent with life. We get confused easily; we tend toward people pleasing and often feel lonely, and our eyes deceive us. Deep down, though, we know there is more to life than what we see in the mirror. We know that we are significant; we're just not sure how.

"I have a lot of faith," writes Anne Lamott. "But I am also afraid a lot, and have no real certainty about anything. I remembered something Father Tom had told me—that the opposite of faith is not doubt, but certainty. Certainty is missing the point entirely. Faith includes noticing the mess, the emptiness and discomfort, and letting it be there until some light returns."[3]

As parents, we often think we have to save our children. That we need to be perfect, so our kids, in turn, become perfect, but that, too, is missing the point. We can't always save them, and we can't always prevent bad things from happening to them, no matter how hard we try. True faith is not found in blessing; blessing, rather, strengthens our faith, so that when the darkness comes, we can run off our faith battery, remembering all the ways God has been good to us. And even though we're going through the valley of the shadow of cancer or death or discouragement, we can know that mountains are ahead—just out of view.

"When we were children, we used to think that when we were grown-up we would no longer be vulnerable," writes Madeleine L'Engle. "But to grow up is to accept vulnerability. . . . To be alive is to be vulnerable."[4]

There is a lot of temptation in the world today—a lot of darkness—and we, as parents, tend to want to shelter our kids from that. We want to create a bubble effect, but the problem with bubbles is that they burst, and then the kid drops, falling hard into the middle of sin and brokenness and despair. Emily's parents tried to create a protective bubble around her, but, like many homeschooled Christian kids, she saw through it. She reached out her hand and popped the soapy film, falling straight into an eating disorder. Not all children will experience hardship when they burst that bubble, but some do. Some lose their way. Others purposely destroy the life their parents try to make for them.

Our children don't need us to fix them. They don't need us to take away the pain. They know we can't. When our little ones scrape their knees, they run to us so we might comfort them. Hold them. Sit in the brokenness and hurt *with* them. This is exhibiting true faith to our children. This is recognizing the limits of our humanity, and the need for the divine. And if we teach our sons and daughters how to feel, and how to sense God's presence in spite of pain, there's less chance of them turning to self-abuse.

When Emily miscarried her first child, she automatically began to restrict her food intake. It wasn't just a muffin, or a sandwich, or a banana. It was distraction, it was salvation; it was mind-numbing hunger so the pain didn't seem so full. She had lost her child. One moment she was carrying him or her or it, and the next moment, the five-week-old fetus was gone, and in its place were a bloody nightgown and a half-eaten muffin.

Maybe it's music, maybe it's cutting, maybe it's drugs, maybe it's over- or undereating, but whatever it is, it isn't the problem. It's a way to avoid the problem, a way to avoid feeling. Eventually, though, the muffin isn't enough, the cutting doesn't cut it, the ice cream doesn't fill us, and we're left emptier for the trying. We need to practice letting ourselves enter the hard places as part of our healing. To know we are very alive for it all. We need to help our children embrace hardship, and to allow our souls to grow by practicing patience and perseverance and joy. We need to teach our young ones to seek out the slivers of light in a roomful of darkness. For pain makes growth possible, and with growth comes hope, and with hope, love. And in the end, it is love we're starving for.

So instead of creating extremes for our children, why don't we embrace the reality of our world, acknowledge that so much of it is not the way it should be, and give our children the tools with which to turn ugliness into beauty? Why don't we equip them with the weapons they need to fight misunderstanding and injustice, weapons like compassion, kindness, goodness, and a desire for justice and humility? To be spiritual in a material world looks odd, different. It means daring to stand up for truth, and this takes courage. It means *making God's thoughts matter more than man's*. And it means helping our children develop the kind of character that prays.

WHAT'S LOVE GOT TO DO WITH IT?

Only when we learn to love ourselves can we truly love our children. After all, being a mom requires a kind of inner strength that rivals that of superheroes. And unless we take the time to nurture ourselves, we will soon run out of the energy and patience necessary to be co-creators.

"The mother-child relationship is paradoxical and, in a sense, tragic," says German philosopher Erich Fromm. "It requires the most intense love on the mother's side, yet this very love must help the child grow away from the mother, and to become fully independent."[5]

Motherhood wakes you up multiple times each night and wipes its snotty nose all over your furniture and commands the attention of mind, body, and soul. Motherhood dies to itself. It is never-ending, and fraught with error, and it is admitting you aren't invincible. It is crying at the drop of a hat and realizing you don't have the virtues you always thought you had. Or perhaps you have heaps more.

And this realization that we cannot physically do everything is one of the healthiest things for reshaping our body image. It reminds us that we are, in fact, mortal, and in need of something more. It helps us to see the truth about our bodies: that they are physical containers for spiritual souls. And unless we take care of our souls, we will not be able to be the life-giving vessels we were created to be. In order to bring life to our homes, our husbands, and our children, we need to rest, to take care of ourselves, to nurture the quiet places.

Some days, we feel the incredible honor of it all, of this molding and shaping little lives, and other days, we don't. On one such day, Emily gripped the sky like a kite, the sky outside her window, desperate for some kind of escape. It was the same sky she looked to when she was in labor, and on this particular day, the birthing pains seared, both children teething and sick with colds and no one sleeping. She stood by the window all cry-eyed and bone tired and wondering at the bigness required of a mother. The strength needed to turn herself inside out, minute by minute, in search of wisdom, empathy, Kleenex, and a lap, and when would it be her turn?

Her twenty-three-month-old Aiden had broken another DVD unintentionally and it had broken her and she had cried in front of him and now he was sobbing in the living room, with her by the window, when baby Kasher began to weep from the swing. It was the same old story of lost perspective, and then she heard it. The hard patter of little feet, running, pausing, running, pausing, and she turned from the window to find her baby with a soother in his mouth, toys piled up and blankets, so many blankets. Aiden was patting Kasher's stomach because he couldn't find his back. And Kasher was quiet.

And she found it. The love that gives perspective. She found it in the heart of her son. A boy who, while sobbing, heard the cries of another, and ran. A boy who brought blanket after blanket, and she realized then that we need not be bigger. We need not be giants of strength. We need only be a child.

OUR MOST ACCURATE MIRROR

We are always learning from our children, even as we try to teach them. We learn amazement, awe, curiosity, genuine concern, compassion, and the ability to make fun of ourselves. Children are a parent's most accurate mirror. It's always shocking to see our facial expressions manifest themselves in our offspring. It's like having little rearviews following us all day long. These reflections make us aware of how we treat ourselves. But this is the kind of mirror we can trust. This is the reflection we want to focus on fixing—the one that presents itself in the lives of our children.

Perhaps your child sighs when she looks in the mirror, or yells at cars on the road, or gets frustrated easily with her siblings and friends. More than trying to tell her how to change, *be* the change. Speak lovingly to yourself when you look in the mirror, bite your tongue when you're tempted to swear at a car, and treat your husband and children with kindness and patience, then apologize when you don't.

There's no doubt about it: it's hard to care for the soul, to let the light in, when society is so full of darkness. It's hard to care about invisible qualities when society tells us we are what we look like. Western culture says we need to have it all together, to juggle countless responsibilities, and to look like models while we're at it. We're expected, as mothers, to hold down full-time jobs, breast-feed our babies, serve homemade meals, and spend quality time with our children, all while satisfying our husbands' needs.

Everyone deals with these pressures differently, but food is the biggest scapegoat. We either "forget" to eat because we don't have time, and then binge when we do, or we snack, not making the effort to have a proper meal. We're constantly feeling guilty because we are trying to please everyone, and meanwhile, our souls are being neglected, and our bodies are becoming empty shells. We need to make time for ourselves. We need to treat ourselves as tenderly as we do our children. To eat, sleep, and live, as though we are carrying life inside of us—because we are. We are carrying ourselves.

"Stop waiting for permission," writes author Sarah Bessey. "Stop waiting for someone to say that you count, that you matter, that you have worth, that you have a voice, that you have a place, that you are called. Stop waiting for someone else to validate the person that you already know you were made to be . . .

"Because, darling, you are valuable. You have worth, not because of your gender or your calling or your marital status or your labels or your underlined books or your accomplishments or your checked-off tick boxes next to the job description of Proverbs 31.

"In Christ, you have value beyond all of that. You abide in love; you can rest in your God-breathed worth."[6]

By accepting this worth, by learning to respect our bodies and throw off any inhibitions, we not only treat ourselves gently, but we also love on our children. Because the loudest examples have no voices.

Mary Pipher offers the following suggestions for how to feel good about our bodies.

1. When you look in a mirror, make sure to notice and remind yourself of what you like about your appearance. This may take some time and practice.
2. When you find yourself being critical of your appearance in the mirror, force yourself to turn away. Say firmly, "Body, you are mine. I like you."
3. Break the habit of comparing yourself to others in terms of appearance.
4. Don't criticize or comment on other women's appearances.
5. Learn to dress comfortably rather than "fashionably."
6. When you meet others, focus on something besides your appearance. Strive to be interesting, nurturing, witty, a good listener, and empathic.
7. Pay attention to the way media depictions of women influence your self-image, and stay away from media that make you feel badly about your body and appearance.
8. Compliment girls and women for other things besides their physical appearance.
9. Learn to value yourself for other things besides your appearance. Keep track of your accomplishments and successes and remind yourself of them often.

10. Develop other interests besides your appearance. Focus on skills or activities that have nothing to do with your appearance.[7]

EMILY'S STORY

I was born into a Christian home. I was taught that God knew me before I was conceived, that I was fearfully and wonderfully made. But all I wanted was to know that my parents loved me. As a girl, I associated God with a very busy man who had creases in his forehead, a man who sighed whenever I asked him for anything.

Compared to many, I had a wonderful childhood. My parents tried very hard to provide for us and to create a nurturing, holistic home. But there wasn't a lot of joy; I don't remember a lot of laughter or warmth or frivolity. Everything was quite serious and scheduled. Love, for my mum and dad, was a peck on the cheek in the mornings, Bible devotions, school lessons at the wooden kitchen table, and a story at night, and it was all good, except for the fact that I didn't *feel* wanted. There was never an intimate talk, never a hug that didn't seem to have to end, never a "please let me hang out with you" moment in which I knew, without a doubt, that I was more than a daily chore.

I was afraid of God because he could send me to hell, just as Dad could ground or spank me, but that was the extent of our relationship. I'd rhyme off a rote prayer each night, then return to planning the next day's meal, and it would be years before I realized God was more than I could ever ask or imagine. It would be years before I learned that the longings in my heart to be seen, heard, and cherished were longings planted in us at birth, longings only the spiritual could fill. As philosopher Blaise Pascal said, "There is a God-shaped vacuum in the heart of every man which cannot be filled by any created thing, but only by God, the Creator."[8]

These longings inside of us—inside our souls—are like map coordinates designed to give us direction, to lead us to prayer and reflection and meditation, because we cannot do this life alone. But I still find myself trying to fill my emptiness by pleasing my children, or eating chocolate, or controlling my waistline, or exercising too long. I look in the mirror, and I see a physical reflection. I don't see a pulsating soul. I see a weary mother who can't even find time to clip her nails. I see a person fraying at the edges for not having time to paint or play guitar or write, all of which define her as a woman. I see my mother.

My mother was always tired. I remember wondering if she was ever happy. I remember wishing she would just sit and drink some tea and laugh with us. That she would dust the flour off her hands and play a game of Monopoly or tell us stories about when she was young or watch a movie. But she didn't have much of a support network, and my father was always working, and because we were always moving, she homeschooled us. Then, there were the bills, which we were always scrimping for, and so she was always worried. If this is what it means to be a Christian, I used to think, I don't want it. Because being a Christian seemed no different, except you had more rules to follow.

But then Mum got brain cancer. She got it hard and long, and for the three hardest years of the tumor, I moved home, at the age of twenty-seven, to take care of her. And she had nothing, not even her mind, but she finally had peace. She was no longer stressed and worried. She'd been emptied, making room for the divine.

"All striving after greater beauty and importance, and greater greatness, is foolishness," writes Lamott. "It is ultimately like trying to catch the wind. Lilies do not need to do anything to make themselves more glorious or cherished. Jesus [says] that we have much to learn from them about giving up striving. . . . He's heartbroken, as when you know an anorexic girl who's starving to death. . . . He's saying that we could be aware of, filled with, and saved by the presence of holy beauty, rather than worship golden calves."[9]

We were all humbled by Mum's illness, by the long stretches of sleeping and incoherence, during which I cried. When Mum was awake, and lucid, we'd sit and have tea and she'd tell me I was beautiful, and because she forgot things easily, she'd tell me this multiple times a day, making up for all the years in which she hadn't. And my dad became a tender and truly loving soul. He stopped going to church so many days a week. He made Mum his new ministry, massaging her feet and changing her Depends. He made me supper and cared about me deeply.

He still does. And, feeling cherished and wanted, I repented for many years of disrespect and dishonor, asking my parents for forgiveness and finding healing in humility. Everything was redeemed: their marriage, our relationship, my faith—it was all made better by something tragic. I couldn't be angry at God for all the sweetness.

Mum was on the cusp of eternity, and she had no more inhibitions. Fear had been extracted from her brain along with the tumor, and this fearlessness made life a gift. Her illness made me notice the small things. It made me thankful for the flit of a sparrow's wing, for our bulging pantry, for the mornings in which she remembered my name. Gratitude—a way of life that makes us believe we are more than our reflection. That we are worth the details in the sunset, the folds of our baby's flesh, the way their skin feels like heaven, the way soil smells after a rain—all these very intentional gifts, put here, on earth, for our enjoyment.

Voskamp puts it this way: "All fear is but the notion that God's love ends. *Did you think I end, that My bread warehouses are limited, that I will not be enough? But I am infinite, child. What can end in Me? Can life end in Me? Can happiness? Or peace? Or anything you need? Doesn't your Father always give you what you need? I am the Bread of Life and My bread for you will never end. Fear thinks God is finite and fear believes that there is not going to be enough. . . . In Me, blessings never end because My love for you never ends. If my goodnesses toward you end, I will cease to exist, child. As long as there is a God in heaven, there is grace on earth and I am the spilling God of the uncontainable, forever-overflowing-love-grace.*"[10]

Since having a miscarriage and watching my first baby wash red from my body, since measuring small with my third, and being put on couch rest; since thirty-six hours of labor in which my body gave way to another and I heard the full-throated yell of Yahweh in nine pounds of infant flesh, I've known a desperate kind of parent love, the kind that would give, and do, anything, the kind that would buy the moon just to see my child smile, and I understand, now, the love of the father God, lavished on us in the beauty of autumn colors and snowcapped mountains and long-necked geese flying south.

REFLECTION

- Do you try to mask pain so your children don't have to suffer?
- How did your own parents teach you to walk through suffering and hardship?
- What is the worst thing that could happen if you simply "let" your child hurt, while holding him, instead of trying to fix the pain?
- What do you personally believe about the meaning of life?
- How do you try to "feed" your children spiritually, each day?

TOOLS

A Spiritual Menu:

- Compassion. It means walking in brokenness with our children so in turn, they'll walk with others. It means being brave enough to just sit, and be, instead of always trying to fix. Help them to see the man on the street begging for food, and take that man for dinner, or make him a sandwich. Say hi to the woman in the wheelchair, and hug the little boy who has no legs. Give your children eyes, that they might see, and a heart, that they might love. In turn, they'll make the world a better place.
- Truth. At dinner, talk about real-life scenarios, about real-life hypocrisy, about real-life hurts; strike up hard conversations with your littles, asking what they think about it all. Then share what you think about it, and plant in them a hunger for truth.
- Prayer. One of the greatest tools you can give your children is the ability to bow their heads and fold their hands and beg for help. Because then, no matter what situation they're in, they will know they are not alone. As Edwin Keith said, "Prayer is exhaling the spirit of man and inhaling the spirit of God."[11]
- Humility. The Bible urges us to do nothing out of selfish ambition or vain conceit, but to consider others better than us (Philippians 2). This trusting our worth, our value, to God, and honoring others before ourselves will grow not only contentment, but love and respect instead of jealousy and competition.

- Gratitude. Create journals in which you and your children in-scribe each night before bed what you're thankful for. Reminding ourselves of the simple gifts such as food, shelter, and family always puts things in perspective.
- Generosity. Teach your children to give—of their time, their energy, and their resources—and then watch as, in turn, you all receive.
- Reflection. It is important to process and engage yourself in thought, to pause and to become better aware and connected to life. Daily devotions can help with this. Numerous books, web-sites, and mobile apps provide daily quotes that are encouraging and supportive. "Thus meditating you will no longer strive to build yourself up in your prejudices, but, forgetting self, you will remember only that you are seeking the Truth," said former New Zealand minister of defense James Allen.[12]
- Community. Creating a community of support and guidance is mandatory. You must have support, not only to survive, but to grow and develop as a person and in your faith. "In a word, live together in the forgiveness of your sins," states German pastor Dietrich Bonhoeffer in his book *Letters and Papers from Prison*, "for without it no human fellowship, least of all a marriage, can survive. Don't insist on your rights, don't blame each other, don't judge or condemn each other, don't find fault with each other, but accept each other as you are, and forgive each other every day from the bottom of your hearts."[13]

LIKE MOTHER, LIKE DAUGHTER

Your Personal Legacy

All women become like their mothers. That is their tragedy.
No man does. That's his.

—Oscar Wilde

WHY WE ARE THE WAY WE ARE

A Mother's Mark

The key to understanding ourselves lies in understanding where we've come from—or *whom* we've come from. For the sake of this book, which centers largely on the female role, we will not be addressing the impact a father's perception of food or body image has on his child—but this is not to discount the incredible impact a patriarch's worldview can have on his family. Nevertheless, "The relationship between mother and daughter probably has the richest potential for emotional closeness of any parent-child bond, along with the greatest potential for disappointment and anger," writes Harriet Lerner.[1]

The first step in understanding yourself is to understand your mother's attitude toward *her*self—and ultimately, her attitude toward food, body image, and physical activity. Emily's self-hatred as a child stemmed, in part, from her mum's shame over her own body. Dena, meanwhile, learned that "fat is bad" (as her mother was always on a diet) and that being overweight makes you miserable. Exploring the impact your mother had on your own body image will offer insight into behaviors that you do automatically. It will help you learn who you are and why you do what you do. Remember, we are not doing these exercises to incite blame, but to encourage freedom by uncovering the truth, to inspire understanding by exploring messages and influences. No matter your relationship with your parents, be fully cognizant of the messages and modeling you received concerning food and body image issues. This will help you to separate the child you were from the adult you've become. "Working things out with your own mother—eliciting her stories and history—is one of the best things you can do for your relationship with your daughter," writes Lerner.[2]

Understanding You

The second step toward understanding where you're at is by evaluating *your*self. We are not our mothers. We may inherit their genes, but how we respond to our children is up to us. Don't be afraid to be firm with the past: tell it to back off while you focus on the present. Then, explore the truth about who you are, apart from who you think you are. This discovery of roots and self is a powerful method for becoming aware of the "why" behind our negative and positive thoughts; it serves as a stepping stone toward breaking free of the past. In turn, new habits and mind-sets can be formed. By embracing the truth about who we are and rejecting the lies, we will be transformed from the inside out. We will radiate the joy and peace and beauty of knowing we are more than our looks. This may not be as easy as it sounds, but working through the issues, recognizing that they exist, and moving forward productively and mindfully will help you to achieve a better understanding of who you are, both in the world and to yourself.

Outside Influences

The third step is to evaluate and explore what the *world* has taught you about your body and food. What have you learned from Western culture, religious traditions, and peers pertaining to body image, food, and physical activity? The media's voice is louder than we realize. Society's airbrushed view of reality bombards us through billboards, magazines, and movie screens. And whether we think we're immune to it or able to wade through the messages, we're more likely to be absorbing those messages subconsciously. It's unavoidable. While it may be hard to determine which messages have come from where, what matters is that you explore *your* story, that you understand which factors have formed your views of body image, self, food, and physical exercise. Where have the messages that you accept as your own come from? Where have they led you?

Finally, realize that you can break free of these views. You can reprogram the messages that have damaged your perceptions, and in turn, form your own opinions. For some, this may mean seeking therapy. For others, it may mean working privately in one's own time to replace those images with new ones. But again, being aware of the messages—those we've incorporated into our lives—is the first step toward correcting and replacing them with healthier ones. After all, you are so much more than what media—or anyone else—says you are.

RETEACHING LOVELINESS

Women are the heartbeat of the home. If we are peaceful, joyful, and confident, our families will most likely be, too. And if we're anxious, fearful, and ashamed, generally our children and husbands will suffer as well. We cannot let our fears of who we *think* we are determine how we parent—fears of passing on insecurities, of saying or doing things that will make our children doubt themselves. Our children will end up being more gracious than we ever thought possible, and not because of us, but *in spite* of us. Because don't most of us, deep down, believe in redemption?

The truth is, we can only believe in redemption once we've experienced it ourselves. And we experience it only when we release our pain, our brokenness, and our emptiness, letting it go. If we keep trying to hold on to our injuries, to damage ourselves further, we'll never be able to fully love on those around us, because our arms will be too full of ourselves. If we accept that we are too fat, too skinny, too short, or too tall, that anything other than what we are is less than good, then we fall victim to the demons and react to them instead of to the world around us.

We need to stop letting fear define us, and to boldly admit we will never be good enough. We need to say, *That's okay, self. Try again another day.* And then, to do our best by our children anyway. To hug them, listen to them, and watch movies with them. To cry with them when their hearts get broken. To let them eat and enjoy it; to let them exercise for fun and good health; to let them indulge every now and again and yet be mindful that food is nourishment first. And further, to eat with them, to break bread and come together to celebrate the fruits of our families, our labors, and our land. Setting a good example for our children is paramount in all areas of life. Our attitudes toward ourselves will be passed on to our children whether we like it or not.

"Remember, your example will last a long time," writes Lerner. "As family therapist Peggy Papp reminds us, the quality of a mother's life and her courage are among her most important legacies to her daughter. 'A woman who can believe in herself when no one else does, who will fight for herself when no one else will, who will continue to struggle even though she is unprotected, this woman demonstrates to her daughter that these possibilities exist.' One great gift a mother can give her daughter is to live her own life as well as possible."[3]

MAKING PEACE WITH THE PAST

And we will mess them up, yes. Every mother messes up her child to a certain degree, for we are all broken. *It's what we do in the mess that matters.* It's how we respond to our fallenness. No one is perfect, not even our children. Our faults may become theirs, and new ones may arise. But when we accept that we are not perfect, and that that is okay, we send the message to our children that it's okay that they are not perfect, and that is okay, too.

"Sometimes [Mom and I] can't communicate well, for no particular reason except that we're mother and daughter and so different," writes Anne Lamott. "I'm so flamboyant and confessional and eccentric, and she's so essentially English, concerned with how things look to others. But she makes me these big pots of soup, and when she leaves, sometimes I cry."[4] This also describes Emily's relationship with her mother. Yvonne is British and prim and proper and would never say "fart," yet Emily goes to the bathroom with the door wide open. But when Yvonne got brain cancer, Emily went home to take care of her. She helped Yvonne to the toilet, she combed her mum's hair, put lotion on her face, and tried to rework the damage the years had done. And when her mum looked at her and smiled with her huge forget-me-not eyes, Emily cried, and it was better than any pot of soup. This reconciliation with our mothers, this learning to understand who they are and where they've come from, this forgiveness of the past is crucial to regaining our sense of self, to finding the strength for paving a new path, and to making peace with our memories.

REDEEMING THE PRESENT

And once we've made peace with the past, we'll find the strength to redeem the present. To laugh at days to come, to savor food like it's a miracle, and to dance with our children. To treat ourselves, and others, with grace.

A friend of Emily's, Michaela, said she used to think about food morning to night. She was so worried about what she weighed and what she looked like that she wasted her life. Now, she says, she lets herself overeat some days. She tells herself, "Oh well, I guess I shouldn't have had that extra doughnut. That's all right. Tomorrow is a new day. I love you, body." In other words, Michaela is learning to accept, and be kind to, herself. In the same way, we need to accept, and celebrate, our children—not just their talents or their beauty, but everything about them: their skin, their length of arm and hair, their stride and stance, their character, their heart, their laugh, their intellect. So they might step out of the house each morning feeling confident and proud, knowing they are cherished simply for *being*.

"My heart is pounding and I can feel it—the impending sense of letting you down," Lisa-Jo Baker writes to her daughter. "How many nights have I whispered into the deep blue of your eyes how beautiful I think you are? . . .

"I am terrified I will get it wrong. I am terrified that here at the beginning of moments in your life that matter I will be at a loss to dress you on the outside with the beauty that lives on the inside. That I will fail this test of mothering a daughter. . . . *And I don't know how to do right by you when it comes to clothes.*

"Why should it matter? I hear myself asking as I toss the short-sleeved gingham pink dress with the tiny cross-stitch flowers aside. Why do I care so much that the white dress with the scalloped edges is too wide around your arms and the onesie underneath is the wrong color?

"Who cares? Who cares? It's just clothing! But it's not. It's years of wondering how the popular girls blow dried their hair so effortlessly and managed to wear jeans that showed off all the right curves, while I drowned in sizes always too big, too awkward, too ordinary on my too thin and bony frame. . . .

"I am desperate to give you a better head start at the race against the world's opinion of women. Your mother will be the one to cement the word 'beauty' into the foundation of who you are so that come the teenage years, come acne and growth spurts, cliques and boys you will not doubt that your beauty is deeper than all of that."[5]

When we punish our bodies for failing to be what we think they should be, our daughters are the ones who suffer. A 2008 study of ninety-one pairs of mothers and college-aged daughters by the Western Oregon University Psychology Division reviewed the effects of maternal eating behaviors and attitudes on girls' eating habits and body image. It also evaluated the effect of the mothers' feedback regarding weight issues, the strength of the mother-daughter bond, the influence of the media, and the mothers' perceptions of their daughters' shapes. Results were based on the girls' body mass index and showed that negative feedback from the mother, maternal disapproval of the daughter's figure, and mothers' eating behaviors and attitudes as perceived by their daughters caused the girls to suffer both in body image and in eating habits. In addition, the study analyzed the daughters' disordered eating scores and found that the mothers' tendencies to internalize media messages regarding thinness and beauty significantly affected the prediction. "Mothers who showed a greater internalization of media messages about thinness were most likely to have daughters with eating pathologies," the study concluded.[6]

Our daughters are watching: they are the ones peering through the cracks in the bedroom door, the ones who catch us changing in the closet or gorging on ice cream or scrubbing away our stretch marks or sobbing on the scales. The ones wondering if to be a woman is to be ashamed. Where is the tender perspective? Where is the grace? To trace our bodies with loving hands and to marvel at the curves that tell our story is to own and love ourselves. To smile into the mirror and watch the crow's-feet land is to reflect on the lives we've led and the paths that have etched their way into our very skin. It is to recognize that stretch marks are the fruits of our literal labor, and the expansion of our bellies the space for our growing babies. Owning our bodies, ourselves, and knowing that every imperfection traces the history of a life lived may help us to accept those areas of our bodies, and ourselves, that are not perfect.

So, women, let's celebrate ourselves. Let's stand proud in our bedrooms and reclaim our womanhood. Let's declare our bodies, in all their nakedness, heaven's glory. For the sake of our children. For the sake of our husbands. For the sake of ourselves.

OUR STORIES

Dena

I am blown away by the honor of raising a daughter and a son. And I'm terrified beyond words of the incredible responsibility. Because raising children is so much more than clothing, feeding, and nurturing them when they are sick. It is an existential process that is transferred from one generation to the other. Some days are easy, and some are a bone-aching challenge. But the good news is, we're not alone. Our parents, and their parents, and countless others before them, all went through this.

This long line of genealogy plays an important role in shaping our views of food, of body, and of self. In this regard, I think it's important to look back at the lessons our parents have taught us. Because no matter how different we are from them, they've shaped us and helped to form our relationship with ourselves.

My mother struggled to accept her body. Growing up, she was always on a diet. As a result, I came to believe that when I got older, I would probably get fat. She never came out and said that to me, but that is how I interpreted her struggle with weight. I learned that fat was not good. I learned that you don't feel good when you are fat, so fat is the enemy. It was also ingrained in me that while I might be beautiful now, I may become fat like my mother when I grow up, which probably means I will be miserable.

So dieting in the home was the norm. The habit worsened in high school, and in college, I began to engage in disordered eating behaviors such as overexercising, binge eating, restricting, and even some purging. I was constantly at war with my body. It was exhausting. I was always battling the curse of being fat. As I grew older and ended the absurd dieting cycles, I began to realize that the war my mother was fighting (and often still fights) was not directed toward me or my body. My mom's conflict with fat and food is about her own discomfort and struggle with body image issues. When I was younger, I took it personally. Even now, it still creeps up on me when I don't expect it, this belief that I am destined to become fat, a belief that in turn makes me feel embarrassed by, and frustrated with, my aging body.

Of course, these body image issues and messages that I received don't negate the fact that my mother was, and is, an amazing mom. I just wish she could see herself more like I see her: as a woman of beauty, love, and grace. Perhaps I should learn to view myself that way too. Thankfully, in recent years, my mom has managed to become more comfortable with herself, to see that life can be enjoyed and not spent following specific protocols for weight loss. As she puts it, "Life is always changing; you just have to accept, and move on."

Emily

Whenever Dad was in the room, Mum would change in the closet. I remember peeking through the door at her white back and slender waist, wondering why she didn't want him to see her, feeling a shame too raw for any nine-year-old to feel, and thinking, so this is what it means to be a woman? And everything in me wanted to cry. For how Mum, in all her beauty, couldn't see herself.

Later I would learn that *her* mother—my grandmother—also hid from her husband because of scars from a childhood disease. And my mum, standing outside the door, saw all of this. My mother was a nurturing woman, a homemaking woman who loved God fiercely but was desperately insecure. She was often afraid, and we, her four children, knew this. We saw fear in the way she handled herself and life—fear of failure, for her father had been a critical man, and her mother was always disapproving. Mum would bake us bread and granola and plan homeschooling lessons and read us *Pilgrim's Progress*, and when we scraped our knees or elbows she would bandage us up. And she told us we were made by a God who loved us, but then we saw the way she got angry when Dad tried to hold her in public, the way she covered herself up and frowned at herself in the mirror. As though it was just too bizarre to think that someone could find her desirable. I imagine she was fighting the voices that had criticized her for years; and she tried desperately to drown them out by memorizing scripture and listening to uplifting music, but it takes years to undo damage done by someone who's supposed to love you.

"It's so hard to get quiet enough, free enough of the bondage of self, to hear the voice in the whirlwind that Job heard," writes Lamott. "There's always so much shouting going on in here. It's a cacophony of sounds from my childhood—parents and relatives and teachers and preachers and voices distilled into what has become my conscience. But I don't think the still small voice is my conscience. . . . It's so hard to hear it though, and sometimes when I think I hear something in my own true voice, I'm so nuts that I'm not sure if it's me or someone pretending to be me. It seems like when it's really you, the voice doesn't even have to talk."[7]

The people who bring us into the world often say one thing (something they wish they believed, and want us to believe) but live another, and I saw this dichotomy in my mother. She spoke of the joy of the Lord, the love of the Lord, yet I rarely saw her laugh, and she seemed happy only when she was in her flower beds. And I always felt so guilty, as though I was somehow to blame for her sadness, not realizing, at the time, that it had nothing to do with me.

We weren't allowed to play with Barbies, or take ballet lessons, or look at fashion magazines. We weren't allowed to watch *The Little Mermaid* because the mermaid was scantily dressed, and we weren't allowed to talk about bodies or bodily functions or underwear. I remember feeling mortified one day when Dad saw my bra hanging off a chair in my bedroom. I could barely look at him for weeks. And so I developed an unnatural fear of the flesh—a kind of deep-rooted shame—and the need to hide my body, as though it wasn't worthy of anyone's attention, whenever possible. I still fight it. I still feel uncomfortable when I'm naked, and my husband is slowly teaching me to trust him with my body, with all its bareness. As though I'm the only woman who's ever had wide hips or a flat chest. As though Trent's not crazy about me, anyway.

My private, English mother has been forced to change over the years. Her brain cancer has made her dependent on others. She knows what it's like to be exposed, to have someone wipe her bottom because she can't, to have Dad wash her in the bathtub, to have me do up her bra. She's had to reveal herself to us, to trust us with her. To make us realize that we need each other. And in turn, we've become a family.

REFLECTION

- How do you and your mother get along?
- How do you and your daughter get along?
- What similarities do you see between the two relationships?
- How do you talk about and/or treat your body in front of your daughter?
- How does your view of yourself match up with what you tell your children about their worth?
- Have you ever apologized to your children? If not, why?
- What do you remember about the mealtimes you had while growing up?

- What messages did your mom send you about body image and self-esteem?
- What messages did your dad send you?
- What were your parents' attitudes toward physical activity?
- How have their opinions shaped yours, and which of them do you actually agree with?

TOOLS

- Tell your children you're sorry for how you've hurt their perception of themselves, and ask them to forgive you.
- Make a list of ways in which you can encourage or positively reinforce your children's sense of purpose and value, and choose a different method each week.
- Seek the therapy or counseling you need in order to be free of the past.
- Create a body image genogram (family tree). This exercise helps make you aware of messages about food, weight, and size that have passed down through generations.
- Time line: develop a time line of when your issues with food, weight, and/or body image issues started.
- List: create a positive and negative list of the attributes, behaviors, or attitudes toward food and body image that have been passed down from generation to generation and that you want to continue or discontinue in your family.
- What self-care behaviors do you use? Which ones are you going to use this week (for example, walk three times, go to yoga class, say nice things when you look in the mirror, listen to uplifting music when driving home from work)?
- What are some of your behaviors related to eating, physical activity, and weight control that you want to change?
- Choose one negative behavior that you're going to stop this week (e.g., pinching your fat, skipping breakfast, talking about needing to go on a diet).

BEING THE MIRROR

How to Inspire Beauty in Our Children

Every time a woman passes a mirror and criticizes herself, there's a girl watching.

—Gloria Steinem

This always being watched creates a lot of pressure. How do we live in a way that inspires beauty? How do we keep our sons and daughters from making the same mistakes? How do we keep them from believing the lies that surround them, the lies that caused us to question ourselves and our own bodies?

As Courtney Walsh, author of *A Sweethaven Summer*, writes, "How do I, with all my disordered eating, a former anorexic/bulimic, train up a girl who doesn't see herself as anything but just right? How big a deal do I make of this to help her see that health is the most important thing? How do I encourage her not to let that feeling of being different stop her from being amazing—from going after the things she's so good at?

"And most of all, how do I make sure she knows she is loved . . . exactly the way she is?

"It's interesting to see your struggles reflecting in the faces of little ones you love so much. And as I talk to her and tell her not to compare herself to other girls . . . and explain that different is good, and it makes us special and unique . . . I wonder if these are the same words God's spoken to me over and over again. . . . The same words I have yet to really hear.

"How do you teach a child to be exactly the opposite of you?"[1]

SEPARATING YOUR ISSUES FROM THEIRS

A common fear that Dena hears regularly in her line of work is, "How do I keep my daughter from developing an eating disorder when I have one?" As a parent, you cannot assume sole responsibility for preventing your child from developing an eating disorder. While there *are* prevention measures and risk factors to consider, your child may still suffer body image issues or weight-related problems. This is not your fault. Diagnosable eating disorders are mental illnesses that have strong hereditary influences as well as environmental factors. The influences behind any one particular eating disorder are extremely complicated and research has not yet shown what combination of factors actually causes an eating disorder.

That said, there are things parents can do to help their children. There are risk factors to look for and steps to take to guide young people. Interestingly enough, the traits that put one at risk for disordered eating (such as a need for control, a sensitive spirit, and an independent mind-set) are, on the flip side, strengths that make one successful. The need for control can develop into efficiency and organization, a sensitive spirit can inspire empathy and compassion, and an independent mind-set can transform into leadership and calling. The parent's responsibility is to channel these traits, to help children flourish in a wholesome and encouraging environment, not to drive them to express themselves in life-threatening ways.

Model Behavior

Though no one is to blame for a person's disordered behavior, it is essential to understand that what our kids see us doing matters. Many habits modeled by mothers, such as dieting, body dissatisfaction, self-criticism and disordered relationships with food, weight, and physical activity encourage children to become sensitive about their own weight.[2] Mothers who criticize and degrade their own bodies subject their children to similar messages about themselves, spoken or unspoken. A recent study spanning a period of ten years showed that ten-year-old children of mothers with disordered eating were more likely to exhibit dietary restraint and overvalued ideas about weight/shape in how they evaluated themselves.[3]

Psychologist Diane Neumark-Sztainer, author of *I'm Like, So Fat: Helping Your Teen Make Healthy Choices about Eating and Exercise in a Weight-Obsessed World*, writes, "Research studies have shown a strong association between the more extreme weight control behaviors in parents and similar behaviors in their teens. . . .

"Many of the eating disorder professionals I've interviewed have told me that, if there's one piece of advice for parents they'd like to see in this book, it's 'Don't diet. Model behaviors you want your children to adopt.'"[4]

But don't just model positive eating habits (such as regular meals, nutritious snacks, and celebrating chocolate and desserts once in a while). Model positive self-esteem, healthy confidence, and complimentary praise. Instead of criticizing yourself in front of your kids, marvel humbly over the use of your limbs, the fact that you have the ability to move, the use of all five senses. Don't comment on a pair of jeans no longer fitting, but instead, put on a loose-flowing dress and twirl around the living room, in freedom and happiness. Notice when your son or daughter or husband makes the effort to look nice; be aware of which comments cause your loved one's face to light up, and make an effort to continue variations of the same compliments over the coming years. It's not easy, this modeling joy and confidence while caring for others, but the more you seek to demonstrate love, the more you'll begin to feel it, too.

A person's self-esteem is her overall evaluation of her worth, taking into account her beliefs and emotions. Healthy self-esteem is armor against the challenges of the world. Those who know their strengths and weaknesses and feel confident about themselves seem to have more resilience handling conflicts and resisting negative pressures. They tend to smile more readily and enjoy life. These individuals are realistic and generally optimistic.

In contrast, individuals with low self-esteem tend to view challenges as sources of frustration. Those who think poorly of themselves have a hard time finding solutions to problems. They tend to take negative situations and internalize them by inferring negative meaning about themselves. For instance, if given to self-critical thoughts such as "I'm no good" or "I can't do anything right," they may become passive, withdrawn, anxious, or depressed. Faced with a new challenge, their immediate response may be "I can't" or "I'm not good enough."

Self- and body-esteem develop from infancy through adulthood. That's why it's important that mothers exemplify healthy self-confidence. It begins by finding balance in your life, with nutrition, physical activity, and weight. There is a relationship between low self-esteem and difficulties with boundaries. Those with low self-esteem tend to be stepped on or used by others because they have difficulty saying no. Thus, it's important to voice what you see, feel, or need by making "I Statements." By expressing thoughts, feelings, and desires in a calm, direct, and honest manner, you show that you are in charge of your life.

It is also essential to both affirm and praise yourself in front of your children. This models confidence and beauty. Be wary of commenting on your weight or body size, as well as remarking on the appearance or girth of others. Challenge your belief about what health looks like. Today's culture promotes a narrow definition of health, and it eliminates the majority of the population that is, in truth, healthy. Thus, we encourage you to start broadening the definition of health and beauty, making it a realistic goal both for yourself and for your children.

Media imaging and advertising can wreak havoc on self-esteem. The whole goal of advertising is to diminish and devalue us as women in an effort to sell products that will ultimately provide us with happiness. We have to guard our minds and protect our eyes. The same is true with Internet sites geared toward capitalizing on girls with low self-esteem. Sites promoting dieting, starvation tips, self-harm, and suicide are dangerous, particularly for those with poor ego strength and low self-esteem.

In addition to protecting our eyes and guarding our minds, we need to cherish our children. We need to give them genuine and varied compliments. Yes, inner beauty is important, but we are often so afraid of vanity that we try to humble the confidence right out of a child. Focus on a few of your son's or daughter's features that are particularly attractive—their soft skin, wavy hair, agile feet, winning smile, or shapely nose. But more than focusing on the physical, remind them of the other features that make them unique: their ability to sing, their caring heart, how hard they try at math and soccer, how kind they are to animals. Remind them of all the things they *do* that make you like them, and of all the things they *are* that make you love them.

Spend time with your children doing things you enjoy; in addition, take interest in the things they love—things that may not interest you, but that set their world alight. And tell them that you enjoy spending time with them, that you are blessed to have them in your life.

Cherish your child. Because we're all just skin-covered souls longing for heaven—longing for a world that has no tears, longing for a place in which we're loved, longing to know that we belong.

The Three Cs

We wish we could tell you the exact recipe for raising children. But we can't. In spite of purchasing countless books on parenting, we still haven't come across one that can answer all our questions about our particular children. It doesn't work that way because there is so much about raising children that books can't tell you. It's a journey that takes us deep within ourselves, in which we learn to relate on a spiritual level with our children—uncovering in us the unconditional love, grace, patience, and wisdom that only God can bestow. It's a journey that provides what we believe are the keys to raising "Beauty-Full Children"— the three Cs, or **Courage, Connection,** and **Commitment.**

Courage

The dictionary describes *courage* as "the state or quality of mind or spirit that enables one to face danger, fear, or vicissitudes with self-possession, confidence, and resolution; bravery." Dena has a shirt she wears all the time that says "Motherhood is not for sissies." She loves this shirt because it reminds her every day as she raises her children that she does it in spite of fear.

As mothers, we make decisions in the best interest of our children. Some are easy and some, extremely difficult, but either way, we step outside of our comfort zones. And we do it in spite of ourselves.

The Wizard of Oz puts it this way: "The courage is already in you"— it is a fearlessness required to withstand the challenges and struggles that raising children brings on a daily basis. Anxiety, life stressors, and everyday challenges can immobilize us as women and as mothers. Dena has met many women who go through life so distracted by fear that they avoid taking any risks or stepping outside of the box. Rather, they are merely going through the motions, disconnected from life.

Set your mind on the fact that this journey called "rearing and parenting children" is going to take a lot of courage—and then yet more courage. This knowing that courage is critical prepares us for challenges and helps set us up for success.

Connection

Without you even realizing it, the challenges of life can disconnect you, not only from your children, but from yourself. Dena counsels many mothers who claim that something—whether alcohol, drugs, anorexia, binge eating disorder, depression, divorce, or loss—has disconnected them from the very things (family, marriage) that fulfill them. When you are disconnected, you simply go through the motions; you forfeit living in the moment. This results in fragmented living, in which you feel like your past is a collection of abstract lines and shadows, and you can't quite make sense of it all. Memories and feelings are vague and foggy. Meaning is lost.

Fostering a mother-child connection is critical in raising "Beauty-Full Children." This is about being able to dial in to your children, allowing them to feel their emotions in an environment that is safe and secure. According to Janet Surrey, a psychologist and professor at Harvard Medical School and the Stone Center, "Learning to tolerate and bear painful or 'unacceptable' feelings in ourselves and those we love is one of the most difficult trials of life and relationships. It is one thing to desire another's happiness; it is another to deny their pain.

"Often, mothers try to defend against or deny their daughter's pain or anger because they have not had a relational context which allows them to know and to act on their own painful feelings."[5]

In other words, it is difficult to tolerate your child's emotions, particularly negative or painful ones, if you do not have space to contain or tolerate them within yourself. It requires a willingness to communicate, but mostly, an ability to listen and feel without judging, deflecting, or negating.

Raising "beauty-full" children is not contingent on your parenting skills, your education, or the success of your career. God made you a mother. God loved you first, so that you could love others, especially your children. But it's important to connect to God's love, not only to feel it yourself, but to show it to your children. Loving children is extravagant if you are connected. Doing special mother-daughter (or son) activities, even something as simple as playing cards, going on a picnic, or riding bikes, can build this kind of bond. It's very easy to get caught up in household chores, work, and our busy schedules. We think we're spending time with them as we drive them to soccer practice or dance rehearsal, or as we work with them on their homework. But truthfully, this type of togetherness doesn't often allow for the intimacy needed to truly open up lines of communication and foster deep connection. It's only when we're intentionally pouring into them that we'll experience the unity, the oneness, the powerful harmony that a family is capable of.

Commitment

Commitment takes on new meaning when you become a mother. The umbilical cord is never truly cut. Upon giving birth, you know that no matter what, you won't let go of yourself or your children. You are in it until you die. As long as you are committed to not giving up, to doing what is best, and to trying again and again, you will make it through. This is commitment. It models "beauty" as well as strength, and through it, you will find purpose, meaning, and value in your life as a woman and as a mother.

Commitment means listening to your child's stories long after bed-time has passed, because she had a hard day and really needs to snuggle. Commitment is making supper, night after night, and doing endless loads of laundry, and sliding notes of encouragement underneath your teenaged son's door because he refuses to talk to you, and getting bruises on your knees from bowing in prayer. Because motherhood is spiritual warfare. We aren't just battling for our children's everyday survival; we're fighting for their souls. So whenever someone tries to diminish the role of motherhood, remember, it's one of the highest callings you could ever have.

Commitment also means taking care of ourselves, so we can con-tinue to take care of our family. *One of the greatest books our children will ever read is our lives.* So when it comes to health, physical activity, and self-esteem, it is worth the "inconvenience" of being healthy, because of the commitment to putting family first. This isn't as easy as it sounds. Some days you won't feel it. You will want to crawl back into bed and say, "Forget it. I can't do this." When those days strike, get up anyway and brush the negative feelings off. Announce, "I am needed, I am im-portant, and I am committed." You may have to repeat this to yourself numerous times. But you shouldn't have to conjure up the strength on your own. No, during this time you need to depend on the support of friends and family. Both Dena and Emily treasure the time they spend with girlfriends sharing the joys and woes of raising a family. These moments spent laughing about or confessing daily situations via texts, Facebook, phone calls, or e-mail can mean the difference between stay-ing in bed and climbing out.

Nurturing and Fostering Identity

Ideally, our sons and daughters will develop normally, without interfer-ence. The goal is to help them establish their identity, separate from their appearance, weight, and size. However, developing an identity in a culture where "image is everything" sets one up for a superficial persona rather than an identity based on substance and heart.

Dena's friend Missy confessed once that because of her curly red hair, she received an enormous amount of attention when she was younger. Everywhere she went, strangers would comment on how beautiful she was. As she got older, however, the compliments became criticisms. She no longer felt special or unique, but rather different, odd, and ugly. At first, losing weight provided the admiration Missy was hungry for. People complimented her, and she felt noticed and valued. Weight loss is highly rated and valued in our society, so this act of dieting provided the affirmation she was looking for.

But then, the dieting turned deadly. It became an obsession with power. Missy could do what most could not—she could starve. It was a feat that required intense discipline. And while others were no longer complimenting her, for she had become dangerously skinny, Missy no longer cared because it wasn't about losing weight anymore. It was about maintaining her identity.

Dieting feels powerful because only a small percentage of the population (0.5–1 percent) becomes anorexic. In hindsight, Missy admitted she had based her worth and value purely on her appearance. Because of her vulnerable temperament, along with the stressor of being teased, she felt food was the only thing she could control. Therefore, being thin became who she was. It became an obsession because the number on the scale was never low enough. The game of weight loss, starvation, and body image distortion is torturous. It turns extremely dangerous when the act of starving becomes more important than eating and, therefore, living.

Since when did size determine worth? Unfortunately, being thin or looking "fit" in this culture says something about us, although this in itself is wrapped in lies and false perceptions. Being thin says that we are loved and accepted. Thus, thin becomes an identity, a way of being, promising deliverance and freedom when in reality, it separates us from the truth.

Separation from these distortions and lies becomes easier when one's identity defers to one's true self and is not solely attached to appearance or weight. We all have people who inspire us. People like Mother Theresa and Martin Luther King Jr., people like Eleanor Roosevelt and Nelson Mandela. And they don't inspire us because of their appearance or size. They inspire us because of their sense of being, of character and faith.

Helping yourself and your children develop a solid understanding of self is crucial in fostering your children's identity. And it starts with being genuine with others, real with your heart, and open with your mind. It's about encouraging self-discovery, uniqueness, and individuality, and bridging those traits with strong values and morals.

Dena loves the poignant part in the movie *The Help* when Aibileen (played by Viola Davis) says to Mae Mobley (the child she nannies), "You is smart. You is kind. You is important." She then asks Mae to repeat this to her. This scene demonstrates identity building in its truest form, helping children to believe in themselves by nurturing inner confidence and self-esteem.

Plus-sized actress Camryn Manheim, author of *Wake Up—I'm Fat!* says, "I think it's a miracle that I laugh every day and walk through my life with pride, because our culture is unrelenting when it comes to large people."[6]

Yet to say that looks are *not* important would be invalidating, both for ourselves and for our children. We need to balance our focus on looks with other redeeming qualities, such as, "I love how thoughtful you are," or "You have a wonderful laugh." Don't put too much emphasis on a single attribute. Kathy Kater, a psychotherapist and author, states in her book, *Real Kids Come in All Sizes*, "Looks are one part of who we are. But the more we remember all the different parts of who we are, the stronger we will be."[7]

Body Image and Media

It comes as no surprise that media have a powerful influence on body image. This is clearly seen in *America the Beautiful*, a documentary by award-winning filmmaker Darryl Roberts that unearths and challenges our nation's obsession with perfection, thinness, and beauty. In a print interview about the film, Roberts said, "One of the main things that made the women in my study feel bad was the pictures of skinny models in fashion magazines. That seemed like a simple fix to me. Just stop reading them if they make you feel bad. They said they couldn't. That's when I realized that women have a love/hate relationship with beauty magazines.

"This is unfortunate, since a recent report states that 70 percent of all women that spend three minutes reading a fashion magazine feel shameful, fat or guilty. It may come as no surprise that most Americans are unhappy with the way they look, but what I wanted to learn was why we're so obsessed with beauty in the first place.

"The concept of beauty is nothing new. It's been around since the beginning of time. What is new is the massive development and power of advertising and technology."[8]

Media's influence via magazine articles, online fashion and entertainment sites, and television presents us with false images, glorified lies, and distortions. How can we base "health" or "beauty" on something that isn't even real? We are letting these fabricated images define our template of beauty. Indeed, recently there has been a backlash against airbrushing photos of women in magazines to remove any blemishes, to shape women into skinnier or prettier versions of themselves. And still there is not enough of this; still the images permeate pop culture.

One mother who was trying to control her daughter's eating habits explained, "I see her gaining weight and I don't want her to have problems when she gets older." Sometimes, as mothers we superimpose our concerns about weight gain, body changes, and body image on to our children. And ironically, our concerns cause our children to harm themselves physically—through eating disorders or otherwise—due to the stress and confusion of it all.

Self-awareness is the first step. We have to separate our personal fears and concerns from those of our children by knowing who we are, along with knowing our weaknesses and strengths, and then consciously realizing that our children are different from us. And vowing, each day, to respect and love those differences, whatever they may be. We cannot live vicariously through our children. But in order to truly do this, and to set our children free to live their lives, we need to accept ourselves. Only then will the inner critic be quieted by a voice that rises up to encourage, champion, and inspire our families.

On a recent business flight, Dena's seat partner, having learned of her profession, began confessing his concerns about his fourteen-year-old daughter. He was worried about her not being attractive, or being made fun of because of her weight. Dena asked the man if his daughter was experiencing weight-related problems when it came to peers, body image, and food. He said no, but he was concerned it might happen. From the father's description, Dena pictured his daughter (seated a few rows behind them) as being on the heavy side. As they deplaned, Dena was able to take a look at her and was shocked to see a completely "normal sized" girl. Dena immediately turned to her seatmate and said, "Your daughter is perfect the way she is. I think *you* have the problem. You should explore why and how her body changes are affecting you."

We need to challenge our own perceptions about weight and body image before we make comments concerning our children. Negative remarks and teasing are much too common in today's homes. Seemingly benign remarks such as, "Are you sure you want to eat that?" or "You are what you eat," as well as blatant discriminatory comments like "fat," "pig," or "lazy" are very hurtful and should be banned. Criticism does nothing to motivate youth. It only inspires self-abuse.

Johnny, one of Emily's foster boys, refuses to wear clothes that aren't cool, that don't look like something Justin Bieber might wear. He's four years old. Four-year-olds aren't supposed to know what's cool. But he does because his biological father makes fun of him for what he wears, and Johnny desperately wants to impress his absentee dad. And every night, no matter how many hugs Emily or Trent gives him, no matter how many times they tell him he's loved, he cries for his mommy. Because no matter our relationship with our parents—no matter how they've hurt or neglected us—it's them we long for when we enter the dark places. It's their approval alone that can bring the light.

So let's be a light for our children. Let's show them the way. Let's hold their hands and point out truths and lies and let's be a constant for them. A source of hope and encouragement in a world that is anything but.

A LETTER FROM MUMMY

Sarah Bessey exemplifies this kind of love in a letter she posted to her daughters on her blog:

Dear Anne and Evelynn:

Here are the lies, my dears:

- You are only as good as you look.
- You are only lovable if you have a rock hard body.
- You can conquer your feelings of inadequacy by being skinny.
- Nothing tastes as good as skinny feels.
- Everyone judges you by how you look and talks about you behind your back.
- Beautiful is defined by your culture (and so it is beautiful to be frightfully skinny with bolted-on boobs and an identi-kit face).
- You are not worthy of love if you are not beautiful.

I'm raising you in a world that thinks you're only as good as you look. And you're being raised by a woman who is still overcoming these lies herself.

The other day, I did an exercise video at home. You were with me, Annie, while the two littles slept and we leaped and kicked our way through jumping-jacks together. "Oh, Mum!" you glowed, "Even your tummy is having fun! Look at it jumping around!" and for a moment, oh, it stung.

I just gave birth to Evelynn two months ago and so yes, my tummy is "jumping around" when I jump around and part of me wanted to sit down and cry for the sudden cacophony of worthlessness and shame that rose up but then you were there.

You were there, looking up at me, having fun exercising and I thought, no. No, I will not cry about how I look in front of you. Instead I told you that this was fantastic and yes, my tummy was having a marvelous time.

When you asked me why we were exercising, I had to lock my lips tight against the "to lose weight because I'm fat because I just had a baby" that threatened to spill out and instead spoke of having fun exercising for energy and playing together to be healthy and strong and hey, later, did you want to go bike riding?

I am looking for the small ways to spare you just a few battles of body-image that seems to strangle and entangle so many of us in the war against women. Like the girls that post their supper every night on Facebook for "accountability" and the ones that over-exercise to punish their own bodies.

The ones that starve themselves and so carve their own flesh with the word "Forgotten" and "Invisible." Like the ones that are apologetic to their husbands because they have a body marked by childbirth. The ones that are terrified of aging. The ones that feel like they are never, no, never not keenly aware of how they look or what they ate or what they will be eating, the ones chained to a scale or a number or a glossy Photoshopped-ideal.

Sure, I will talk and teach and train but I am learning this: you will sing my songs.

And so I will sing a song of wonder and beauty about womanhood for you to learn from my lips.

I will lead the resistance of these lies in our home by living out a better truth.

I will not criticize my sisters for how they look or live, casting uncharitable words like stones, because my words of criticism or judgment have a strange way of being more boomerang than missile, swinging around to lodge in your own hearts.

I'll wear a bathing suit and I won't tug on it self-consciously. I will get my hair wet.

I will easily change my clothes in front of your Dad, proud of my stretch marks that gave us a family, of breasts that nourished his babies.

I will prove to you that you can be a size 12 and still be sexier than hell.

I will prove to you that you don't have to be all angles and corners, that there is room for some softness because you all love to hug on my soft bits, burrowing into my arms and my breasts to rest for a while.

I will eat dessert and raise my glass and laugh my way to deeper smile lines.

I will celebrate your own beauty, my tall girls, but I will do my best to praise your mind, your heart, your motives, as much as I praise your beauty.

I will not let the words "I'm fat" cross my lips—especially in front of you, my beautiful girls.

I will celebrate beauty where I find it, in a million faces uniquely handcrafted by a generous God with a big tent of glorious womanhood.

I will tell stories of women and surround you with a community of women who are smart and strong, crazy and hot-headed, gentle and kind, women who love and you will see that this is what is beautiful, that a generous love is the most gorgeous thing you could ever put on.

I love you.
Mummy[9]

REFLECTION

- How do you seek to cherish your daughter? To let her know she is worthy of respect? That she is more valuable than her looks?
- How do you talk about yourself in front of your children? Do you strive to set an example in body image, self-esteem, and perspective?
- What kinds of media and messages do you allow in your home? How do you think these are affecting you and your children?
- Do your children know that you love them? Do they know that you love your husband? Do they know that you love yourself?

TOOLS

Promote a Healthy Environment

- Talk openly, listen, and be creative in solving problems.
- Organize family mealtimes.
- Watch your attitude toward eating, drinking, drug use, and handling stress.
- Monitor and curb talk about your own body and the bodies of others.
- Challenge beliefs about thinness, exercise, dieting, beauty, and so on.

Make 'Em Media Wise

1. Teach media literacy. Point out that advertisements have two purposes:
   a. To use the power of persuasion (to get your attention)
   b. To make money

2. Reduce media exposure.
   a. Limit television, magazines, and computer time.
   b. Forbid teasing about weight or making negative body comments in the home.
   c. Teach your family to question the purpose of media:
      • What do you like and/or dislike about this show?
      • Who are your favorite characters? Why?
      • What qualities do you see in them? Strengths, beauty, smarts?
      • How do you know they have these qualities?
3. Increase awareness of media distortions and media messages. YouTube has great videos to demonstrate how models are airbrushed for magazine covers.
4. Look for positive examples in our culture of health and beauty based on attributes other than appearance and weight.
5. Don't be a consumer of the media if you don't agree with it!

Regular Eating

1. Don't diet. If you need to make changes to your weight because of health, focus on behaviors, not weight. Look at how you and your family are out of sync in regard to nutrition and physical activity.
2. Follow the guidelines for intuitive eating, listed in chapter 7, including:
   • All foods fit
   • No "good" foods, no "bad" foods
   • Balance, variety, moderation

Improve Body Image

• Focus on the body's functions; identify three positive attributes about yourself including things about your body.
• Give yourself compliments in front of your children.
• Redefine "beauty" and "health" in your home.
• Talk about balance, variety, and moderation.

- Teach that bodies come in all shapes and sizes.
- Talk about normative body changes.
- Emphasize function over form.
- Show that advertisements lie.
- Encourage nurturing the body with compassion.
- Obtain adequate sleep and quiet time.
- Show body pride—good posture.
- Wear comfortable clothing.
- Challenge negative thoughts.
- Do not make negative comments about yourself, especially about your weight and appearance.
- Do not make negative or positive comments about others regarding weight, such as, "Oh you look so good, you've lost weight."
- Go on family outings that involve physical activity.
- Take teasing and bullying seriously.
- Develop a "no-tolerance" zone at home.
- Help youth differentiate between when to tell an adult, when to walk away, and when to say something back.
- Teach kids how to "shrug it off."
- Teach them how to "throw others off."

Promote Overall Self-Esteem

- Establish eye contact.
- Develop special talents.
- Promote valuable relationships and role models.
- Learn self-soothing and balancing methods.
- Create a personal mission statement.

THE ANXIOUS MOTHER

Using Food, Exercise, or Work as an Escape

Anxiety does not empty tomorrow of its sorrows, but only empties today of its strength.

—Charles Spurgeon

So this is motherhood, with all its tears and begging for wisdom and wanting our children to grow tall while keeping them small forever. It's a letting go and a drawing close, a disciplining and motivating, a praising and correcting, and such a fine balance.

"Through the blur, I wondered if I was alone or if other parents felt the same way I did," writes Debra Ginsberg, author of *Raising Blaze: A Mother and Son's Long, Strange Journey into the World of Autism*, "that everything involving our children was painful in some way. The emotions, whether they were joy, sorrow, love or pride, were so deep and sharp that in the end they left you raw, exposed and yes, in pain. The human heart was not designed to beat outside the human body and yet, each child represented just that—a parent's heart bared, beating forever outside its chest."[1]

From the moment we awaken—toddlers dumping oatmeal on heads and babies pulling toilet paper from the roll—until night, when they're running naked after bath and we're counting the minutes until bed, it can feel uncontrollable. Unpredictable. Overwhelming. Not only are we reminded of issues we had with our mother as we stare at her features on our daughter, or of the way we haven't spoken to our father in years, but we're faced with our own mortality, with the fact that we don't know ourselves as well as we'd like to, that we don't know what to teach our children about joy and life and love. From day to day it can feel hard—there's grocery shopping, cleaning, working if we have a job, getting kids to school and to activities, paying the bills, picking up the dry cleaning, exercising, eating, and showering, not to mention maintaining some kind of social life. Modern life has no shortage of demands on our time, and finding time to care for ourselves, and our families, can be difficult, even on good days. Mothers often tend to martyr themselves in light of others' needs—grabbing a handful of popcorn for lunch on the run, or a roll on the way to dropping children at school, or forgetting altogether to eat and nourish themselves. When you couple all this with a predisposition toward disordered eating or poor body image, it's easy to see how one could slip into the abyss of an actual disorder, and if not that far, then certainly into the realm of low self-esteem and poor self-acceptance. We end up treating others poorly, yelling at the kids, lashing out at our husband, and then abusing food because we feel so ashamed of our behavior.

During these times, it's essential that we become mindful of such slippages, and correct them as they start to wind out of control. We *can* sit and eat a meal with our children, and if they are demanding more milk or a different fork or a different dinner altogether, it's okay to say, "No, Mommy is sitting down now to eat; when I am done, if you still need more milk I will get it for you." It is okay to ask a husband to grab extra items for the table. It's okay to order in. The point is that sitting and eating, and taking time to care for our bodies, is an essential part of being a parent. It's not enough to tell children they need to eat and exercise; modeling it for them is just as important. We may think they don't see us sneaking that handful of chips instead of eating dinner, but they do. We may think they don't notice when we miss a meal, but they do. And the message those actions send is worse than saying, "You can wait a minute for me to take care of myself."

When life seems overwhelming, when you feeling like you might be teetering on the edge of some precipice of self-denial, it may be helpful to

- be mindful of the situation;
- take stock of what is going wrong to prevent you from caring for yourself;
- allow some things to remain "undone"—for example, the laundry can wait a day;
- pray, meditate, or go for a walk to gain some perspective and peace;
- talk to a friend, your husband, a therapist, or your doctor;
- remind yourself it's okay not to be perfect;
- hug your kids and let them know that even though they didn't get that special fork or spoon tonight, you'll try to remember tomorrow, but you really enjoyed having dinner with them.

Strangely enough, when we take time to just sit and rest, life with all its problems becomes more bearable. The quiet voice of calm becomes audible. And love becomes more possible. Because this much is true: life is short, and there should be time to love. You can't go wrong if you love somebody. And the more you love somebody, the more you die to yourself. And death isn't scary. It's probably the most beautiful thing in the world.

SYMPTOMS OF AN ANXIETY DISORDER

Some days, the other voices are too loud—the ones that make your nerves taut and your muscles ache, the ones that shout of stress and fear and insomnia and worry.

Anxiety disorders are the most common mental illness in the United States, affecting five million children and teens, and forty million adults aged eighteen and older.[2] From the age of fourteen (around puberty) until fifty, a female is twice as likely to have an anxiety disorder as a male.[3] Defined as a group of mental disturbances characterized by anxiety as a central or core symptom, an anxiety disorder is more than an anxious feeling. Rather, it's a condition associated with a wide range of physical illnesses, medication side effects, and other psychiatric disorders. Anxiety disorders influence the functioning and quality of life and lead to costly medical workups, negatively impacting one's overall health and well-being. Specific forms of the disorder include:

- Panic disorders, such as agoraphobia, which are defined by the fear of places or situations in which an individual might suffer from a panic attack.
- Phobias—that is, a severe and irrational fear of specific objects or situations, compelling the individual to avoid them. Social phobias are characterized by a fear of humiliation, judgment, and scrutiny, and manifest themselves through an avoidance of public performance.
- Obsessive-compulsive disorder (OCD), a common disorder affecting 2–3 percent of society and defined by persistent and intrusive thoughts or images that accompany compulsive and repetitive behaviors, OCD can be debilitating, agonizing, and significantly disruptive to the individual's functioning.
- Stress disorders, including post-traumatic stress disorder (PTSD) and acute stress disorder, are reactions to traumatic events in an individual's life.
- Generalized anxiety disorder (GAD) is the most commonly diagnosed anxiety disorder, and it frequently occurs in mothers and young adults.[4] The most characteristic feature of GAD is worry, which tends to be intense, prolonged, and uncontrollable. For example, if you worry about your weight, food, the economy, and your finances for hours each day; if you can't perform your usual tasks, have difficulties sleeping, and are aware that your fears are irrational, these symptoms may be indicative of GAD. This diagnosable disorder is a mental illness, and differs greatly from

everyday anxiety or stress. Individuals with GAD are not triggered by a specific situation. Life stressors such as the economic downfall do not need to happen for someone to have GAD. Rather, those with GAD don't know how to stop the worry cycle because it feels beyond their control.

As mothers, we must become aware of our fears and learn to manage them. Anxiety is a natural reaction to stressful and uncertain situations; it is our body's way of telling us to stay alert and protect ourselves. It often serves as a motivator to watch our children, pay attention to our spending, save for an emergency, work to keep our jobs, or consult a trusted financial expert. However, a person may have bigger problems (and a diagnosable anxiety disorder) if her fear becomes so severe she is not able to function. Anxiety disorders run in families and have a biological basis much like other mental illnesses. They develop from a complex set of risk factors including genetics, brain chemistry, personality, and life events. In light of the fact that anxiety disorders frequently

Table 11.1.   Is this everyday anxiety or an anxiety disorder?

Everyday Anxiety	Anxiety Disorder
Worry about paying bills, landing a job, a romantic breakup, or other important life events	Constant and unsubstantiated worry that causes significant distress and interferes with daily life
Embarrassment or self-consciousness in an uncomfortable or awkward social situation	Avoiding social situations for fear of being judged, embarrassed, or humiliated
A case of nerves or sweating before a big test, business presentation, stage performance, or other significant event	Seemingly out-of-the-blue panic attacks and the preoccupation with fear of having another one
Realistic fear of a dangerous object, place, or situation	Irrational fear or avoidance of an object, place, or situation that poses little or no threat of danger
Making sure that you are healthy and living in a safe, hazard-free environment	Performing uncontrollable repetitive actions such as excessive cleaning or checking, or touching and arranging
Anxiety, sadness, or difficulty sleeping immediately after a traumatic event	Recurring nightmares, flashbacks, or emotional numbing related to a traumatic event that occurred several months or years before

Source: Anxiety and Depression Association of America (www.adaa.org).

coincide with other illnesses (i.e., OCD, panic disorders, social phobia, depression, and sleep disorders), it is important to raise any concerns you may have with your doctor, who can make a proper referral to a therapist specializing in your area.

TREATING GAD

Anxiety disorders can be effectively treated with psychotherapy, medication, or a combination of the two. Cognitive behavioral therapy, or CBT, teaches skills for handling anxiety, which help those with GAD learn to control their worry. Some find that medication is helpful; the U.S. Food and Drug Administration has approved several antidepressants for the treatment of GAD. There are also alternative ways to manage anxiety such as relaxation techniques, yoga, or exercise. If you struggle with GAD, we'd encourage you to talk to a psychiatrist and a therapist about the options you have for managing your anxiety. A psychiatrist will help with medication options, while a therapist will work with you through the mental and emotional anguish of the disorder.

AN ANXIOUS ERA

Let's face it: these are fearful times. Witnessing today's economic horizon, not knowing who to trust either online or in the real world, trying to hold down a job while finding a man of integrity to marry, and fretting about how to pay the bills are just a few of the debilitating stressors that affect women today.

In fact, worries about finances have long been a leading cause of anxiety for Americans. In a recent poll conducted online by the Anxiety Disorders Association of America, 45 percent of respondents revealed personal finances to be their greatest stressor.[5] Jenny, a forty-three-year-old woman, became so anxious about money that she ate mindlessly all day. Sometimes, she told Dena, she would eat meals that she later would not remember. She would find empty wrappers and boxes she had no memory of opening. Mortgages, private school tuition, and bills had become such a concern that her weight was significantly affected. Having put on twenty-seven pounds in five months, she felt ashamed, embarrassed, and even more anxious.

We don't all overeat when we're anxious. Some of us undereat. Some of us feel we physically can't pick up a fork or open the fridge, and others of us open it far too easily. Similar to the childish belief that we have a dessert stomach and a meal stomach, we also have a spiritual stomach known as our soul. It is a stomach that is aching for spiritual nourishment, but we often try to fill it with food when it can be filled only by prayer, inspirational readings, music, rest, community, and faith.

Nevertheless, in a world full of sex predators and child molesters; in a world with twenty-four-hour news and bombings and accidents and the threat of nuclear war, anxiety is as physical as a headache, and we tend to try to fix it physically, too. We go to the gym instead of to church; we eat a bucket of fried chicken instead of bowing to pray; we yell at our children instead of putting on some upbeat music and dancing with them. But the more we recognize that anxiety is a spiritual and emotional issue, and the more we tend to it as such, refusing to allow it to rule our lives, the greater the calm we will feel, and in turn, the greater the calm our children will feel.

Studies have shown that anxiety not only harms the patient; rather, it harms those in the care of the patient. So if a mother is feeling stressed, her children will also internalize those feelings. According to Dr. Allan Schwartz, LCSW, "The problem with the anxiety disorder is that everyday life is experienced by the anxious person as dangerous in the absence of any real threat."[6] Schwartz says that studies have proven how anxiety affects a mother's behavior toward her children. These behaviors include:

1. Guilt to control the children's behavior
2. Possessiveness to keep the children close
3. Low expressions of affection from the anxious mother to the child
4. Overall poor communication skills toward the child

An irrational fear of strangers, society, and objects can cause mothers to stunt their children's social growth. Not wanting their children to be hurt in any way, and hoping to somehow protect them from these imaginary threats, an anxious mother can in fact keep her child from becoming independent and autonomous, thereby breeding fear in future generations.

TIGER-MOTHER ANXIETY

In addition to all the other types of anxiety disorders, there's Tiger-Mother Anxiety. A term recently coined after the release of Yale professor Amy Chua's book *Battle Hymn of the Tiger Mother*, Tiger-Mother Anxiety is the pressure to form Ivy League children before they reach the age of five.

"The Asian tiger mom that Amy Chua portrays in her new book may seem like just one more species in the genus Extreme Parent—the counterpart to the hovering American *Parenshelicopterus* or the Scandinavian Curling Parents, who frantically rush ahead of their children, sweeping their paths clear of the tiniest obstacles," writes Nancy Gibbs in her *Time* magazine article, "Roaring Tigers, Anxious Choppers." "The common characteristics include an obsession with a child's success, a reflex to treat kids as extensions or reflections of oneself and patterns of conduct that impartial observers might class as insane if not criminal, if not both. In Chua's case, this famously includes prohibiting grades lower than an A, TV, playdates and sleepovers, and warning her pianist child that 'if the next time's not PERFECT, I'm going to TAKE ALL YOUR STUFFED ANIMALS AND BURN THEM.' In the case of the classic Western helicopter parent, it starts with Baby Einstein and reward charts for toilet training, and it never really ends."[7]

Needless to say, the pressures on mothers are enormous in this culture. We are pulled in countless directions and often don't know how to negotiate everything there is to get done. "American parenting is child-centered, expert-guided, emotionally absorbing, labor-intensive, financially expensive and is expected to be done by mothers alone. And it is impossible to do alone," writes sociologist Sharon Hays. "The mothering you see today in America is culturally and historically unprecedented. We expect selfless devotion to what we interpret as the child's needs, wants and interests at every moment of the day. And with the vast majority of mothers working, that puts them in an impossible paradox."[8]

Many of us walk around in a state of panic not even knowing we are anxious. It has become an ordinary state of being. We experience tightness in our chest and tension or knots in our shoulders and stomach; we have difficulty sleeping and feel overwhelmed on a daily basis and think of this state as normal. In an attempt to control our haywire emotions, we monitor our food intake (or don't monitor it enough), overexercise (or don't exercise at all), and develop weight-related problems. Body image issues become an outlet for anxiety. Several studies have shown that the onset of anxiety disorders precedes the development of anorexia nervosa and bulimia nervosa.[9] The prevalence of OCD, in particular, is much higher with cases of anorexia and bulimia than in a nonclinical group of women in the community.[10]

Laura, age thirty-six, rises at 5 a.m. every day to run eight miles; then, after taking the kids to school, she exercises for six more hours. Her body has become so compromised with injuries that she's been forced to have knee surgery. She is ruled by the fear that if she stops exercising, she will gain weight.

Shari's anxiety began at sixteen when she lost her father to cancer. After she had children, the disorder was exacerbated to the point that she became immobile. She describes her anxiety as a dark cloud closing in on her. Some days she feels like she's suffocating.

LISTENING TO THE WHISPER

Perhaps you're someone who is laid back and relaxed and lets the neighborhood kids tramp mud across the floor. You don't let a lot get to you, or you bottle things up so others can't tell they're getting to you.

Or maybe you are a sensitive, gentle soul who gets stressed out by mud on the linoleum. Who longs for perfection and suffers intensely from past hurts and disappointments. You are easily overwhelmed by people and expectations, and you turn to food, exercise, and/or work to distract yourself from the fact that you're not the woman you want to be, or the woman you feel you need to be, in order to satisfy other people.

And now you're a mother and you're intensely in love with this miniature you. You want her to treat herself with the utmost kindness, and yet you teach her (silently) to starve herself all day and then binge every evening. Because she notices what you to do to yourself.

Your fear of never being good enough controls you. And no amount of reproduction will actually reproduce another you. It takes something more to be born again, to become a woman whose mental strength is not determined by her surroundings. It takes choosing to believe in love, and loving yourself. It's the good angel versus bad angel scenario. Will you listen to the loud voice of condemnation that tells you you'll never amount to anything, a voice that reflects all the lies you've ever believed? Or will you hear the quiet one, the whisper, the holy hush that tells you that you are someone special? Someone unique?

It's easy for us as mothers to think we'll never be good enough for our children, or for us as wives to think our husbands deserve someone better, but this is just a trick to get us to stop trying. Because our husbands fell in love with us, once upon a time. And we may not be perfect mothers, but we're perfect for our children. They need us, desperately. And so instead of living under the weight of self-judgment, let's shower ourselves with grace.

When you start listening to grace, and believing it is true, the lies will slowly dissipate until what you're left with is the reality that you are loved. Your skin, stretching across bone and muscle and curve, is canvas, and your mobility, your vitality, your breathing in and out and in and out is a picture of beauty. Your body is the vessel that holds your soul, and your soul is beautiful, so how could its package not be, too? Our physical imperfections don't define us; we see them more acutely than others do, and if we remember that there are eyes looking at us with love, we can remember that we deserve that love.

Emily has led body image seminars for campers at RockRidge Canyon, a Young Life camp for teenagers, and during those seminars she looks out at a roomful of confused and lonely girls and urges them to speak love to themselves. Specifically:

1. When you hear a voice telling you that you're ugly or not worthy of food or a big mistake, tell yourself out loud that you are beautiful. Look into the mirror and say, "I love you, body. I love you, arms. I love you, legs." And every time you speak love to yourself, it will become easier to believe.

2. Remember that we are all broken, and when someone says something unkind to you, they are most likely just feeling unloved themselves.

3. You were born with a purpose. You are here to change the world in your own unique way. The mirror provides a distraction from that purpose. Those negative voices want to dissuade you from making a difference. Don't let them. Discover your gifts and your talents, and use them to help others.

4. If you struggle with eating, and want to get well but don't feel like you can, don't look at the big picture. Don't look at a full plate of food. Rather, just pick up the fork and take a single bite at your next meal. And at the meal after that, take two bites. Small steps lead to great victories.

5. You cannot control what others think about you, but you *can* control how you think about yourself. However, it takes practice. It takes hard work to separate your opinion of yourself from the opinions of others. So don't give up. Every time you have a negative thought, counter it with a positive one. And pray that your perspective of yourself, and of others, will be reshaped into a vision of love.

Listening to a voice so quiet you have to silence the world takes discipline. In time, though, this voice will become your shepherd, guiding you home.

REFRAMING/RESTRUCTURING THOUGHTS

Listening to this voice requires you to reframe your thoughts. Following are some tips for how to take back your mind and your soul from the stress that surrounds you.

Empowering Coping Thoughts

- I am tired of anxiety/OCD ruling my life. I want to change.
- That's just my OCD talking again. Be quiet, OCD!
- Worried thoughts are not truths. They are lies.
- I do not *have to* act on these thoughts, even though it feels like I do.

Rational Coping Thoughts

- These thoughts are not reality based even though they feel very real.
- If I do my compulsive behavior again, then I will feed the addiction.
- The only way to overcome my fears is to face them. The more I face my fears, the less scary they become.

Healthy Coping

- Obsessive thoughts do not just go away.
- Compulsive behavior lowers anxiety in the moment but worsens it in the long term.
- Compulsive behaviors are negative reinforcement.
- Facing our fears is the way to overcome OCD/anxiety.
- Short-term pain for long-term gain.

EMILY'S STORY

There is no greater humility than that of being a mother. Found there in the low light of afternoon, rocking, one on each hip, while the three of us shed tears and me, mustering strength to be the bigger person.

He's been screaming for the past forty-five minutes, this toddler. Half an hour in nursery at coffee break, and then the entire wagon trip home, and I feel sad for him, and embarrassed by him, and angry for the way I longed for that time to myself, that time of discussing the Psalms with other mothers, and why God allows bad things to happen.

And he feels the Psalms so deeply today, this screaming child, even as we arrive home, and he stomps his tiny foot and I don't know whether to hug him or discipline him. How I wish he could talk. Put these feelings into words, and even as he learns the words, to name his emotions.

And then my three-month-old begins. So we sit and we rock, two crying babies in the low light, the house undone and the world off-kilter. And I remember days of quiet. Days when I could do anything I wanted. Days empty for the filling, and now, four arms and legs and two faces beg my devotion and I don't know how to keep on.

But it happens in the blue whisper of spirit, and I speak to my oldest son now, remind him of God's being bigger, of Christ's living in his heart, and I point to his heaving chest and tell him he has nothing to be afraid of, this child with the bleeding soul. And he nods and says, choking, "God."

And we rock. We sit and we rock while the house needs a vacuum and the dishes pile high. We rock while books and assignments remain unwritten. We rock until their cries subside.

And it's the hardest job in the universe and such an important one, and we never stop carrying them, these babies, and their weeping makes our wombs ache. And sometimes all we can do is hold them in the afternoon, while God sings his love over them.

At thirteen, I was told I couldn't have children. At twenty-three, I told my husband I didn't want to have children. At twenty-nine, I decided I did, and then I miscarried.

This was followed by foster-care training, a failed adoption, and finally, the conception of our son, Aiden Grey. Today, we not only have two sons of our own—Aiden Grey and Kasher Jude—but two foster boys as well, and all of this is something I would have never imagined, me never having wanted children.

And it's been the most anxiety-filled ride of my life, this giving birth and taking care of and loving on our children. But I am learning to listen to a voice that tells me I am beautiful even when I have spit-up on my shirt and infant cereal in my hair and poop on my hands. It's a voice that is becoming louder than the one that tells me I don't belong.

Louder than the one I trained my ears to hear as a young, insecure girl seeking control and identity; louder than the one that lured me into a false sense of self through calorie counting and weigh scales and obsessive exercise.

Now, when I am rocking all four of my babies on the floor, or one is screaming at the other and the other two are flinging food and the world seems like a giant zoo and I have deadlines to meet and dinner to cook and phone calls to answer, I walk into my soul and sit down and rest for a while. I take time to hear the whisper of peace that reminds me, *people are eternal.* They are worth investing in. These children are worth serving. They are my number-one ministry, and one day, they will thank me. For putting aside *me,* so I can focus on them. For taking care of me, so I can better care for them. For learning to love me, so in turn, I can love them.

Their beds were ready. I'd bought the boys blankets—the fuzzy kind that makes you feel like you're being hugged while you sleep. And I'd bought one for Aiden, too, because he would notice, and I need to be extra careful about that kind of thing. About the way he sees, with his old-soul eyes.

Trent would be picking up our foster sons from their mother's in an hour, and then it was a two-hour ride to our hamlet and I couldn't stop thinking about the day they first came here, over a month ago. Holding each other's hands and looking so very small. It had been one of those weeks of wrestling with the angels. Of exercising on the elliptical while listening to music and weeping. Praying one night for these children coming, and the next night for my own boys, and all of them under four, and wondering if we were doing the right thing in offering to take care of my friend's kids.

I can't explain the love I feel for them. I feel like the shepherd in the Bible who risks the lives of his ninety-nine sheep so he can bring the one (or two, in our case) home, and trusting that the rest of the flock will be protected in the meantime. And slowly, I—an obsessive-compulsive disordered eater—am learning to let go. To step into a place that is entirely uncontrollable, the most fearful kind of place I could ever have imagined, and to be at peace. With myself, with my thoughts, with my family, and with my God.

REFLECTION

- Are you constantly worried about what others will think, about the safety and well-being of your children, and/or about whether or not you have enough money? Does anxiety run your life?
- Can you remember a time when you weren't anxious? If so, when or why did things change?
- Are you happy? If not, why?
- What kind of inner voice do you listen to—is it critical or loving?

TOOLS

Managing Anxiety and Stress

When you're feeling anxious or stressed, these strategies will help you cope:

- **Practice mindfulness.** Be in the moment, nonjudgmental, one thing at a time.
- **Take time.** Listen to music, get a massage, or learn relaxation techniques.
- **Eat well.** Remember balance, variety, and moderation. Do not skip any meals or diet. Keep healthful, energy-boosting snacks on hand.
- **Limit caffeine**, which can trigger anxiety and panic attacks.
- **Go to sleep.** When you are stressed, your body needs additional sleep and rest.
- **Move your body.** Daily exercise helps you feel good and maintain your health. Check out the fitness tips on the next page.
- **Remember to breathe.** Take deep breaths. Inhale and exhale slowly.
- **Do your best.** Instead of aiming for perfection (which isn't possible), be proud of yourself for trying your best.
- **Accept.** You cannot control everything. Put your stress in perspective. Reframe.
- **Welcome humor.** A good laugh goes a long way.
- **Maintain a positive attitude.** Make an effort to replace negative thoughts with positive ones.

- **Get outside yourself**. Get involved. Volunteer or become active in your community; not only does this provide a support network, it also gives you a break from everyday stress.
- **Learn your triggers**. Is it work, family, school, or something else you can identify? Write in a journal when you're feeling stressed, and look for a pattern.
- **Talk to someone**. Tell friends and family you're feeling anxious and overwhelmed, and let them know how they can help you. Talk to a physician or a therapist for professional help.

Physical Activity Tips: Stay Healthy, Manage Stress

To get the most benefits from exercise, try to include at least two and a half hours of moderate physical activity (e.g., brisk walking) each week, one and a quarter hours of vigorous activity (such as jogging or swimming laps), or a combination of the two.

- **Find joy in movement**. It's important to discover forms of exercise that are fun or enjoyable. You do not have to run thirty minutes on the treadmill if that is not enjoyable to you. Planting a garden, playing Frisbee with your kids, and going for a bike ride are a few activities that get your body moving and have positive benefits.
- **Set small daily goals** and aim for consistency rather than quantity. It's better to walk every day for fifteen to twenty minutes than to wait until the weekend for a three-hour fitness marathon.
- **Schedule your physical activity**. Make it a priority. You are worth the effort it takes to be healthy.
- **Find a partner**. Connect with an "exercise buddy." It's often easier and more enjoyable to stick to your exercise routine when you do it with a friend, partner, or colleague.
- **Be patient**. It takes time to get into a routine. And even after you get into a routine, you'll have "off" days or weeks—but be gentle with yourself. It's a process. And the goal of it all is not to get stricter with yourself, but to love on yourself more fully.

FRIENDLY COMPETITION

Your Relationship with Other Women

She is a friend of mind. She gather me, man. The pieces I am, she gather them and give them back to me in all the right order. It's good, you know, when you got a woman who is a friend of your mind.

—Toni Morrison, *Beloved*

MOTHER TO MOTHER

It is only natural to compare ourselves, to notice what someone else looks like, talks like, lives like, but it's when we take it to the next level, when we say that this person is better or worse than us because of A, B, or C, that we sin against ourselves and against them. And then there's labor, and delivery, and the baby weighing in at so-and-so, and measuring such-and-such, and relatives making comments, and us feeling worried because our child isn't living up to other people's standards. It's funny, but eventually every child (except those with genetic, developmental, or chromosomal disorders) ends up walking, talking, eating solids, and going to the potty. We're just not good at waiting because we stress about our neighbor's kids instead of championing our own.

We also compare ourselves in terms of how quickly we fit back into our jeans compared to other moms (and worse, to celebrities). We look at our bodies and wonder how THAT mom got in shape so quickly while we still have soft middles and saggy bottoms. Mommy blogs, reality shows, and fashion magazines feed the fire of competition; they objectify women and make it easier to sabotage one another in the name of power and glory. In the end, we're all covered in mud. It's so easy to hurt someone else when we're feeling unappreciated or unaffirmed. To criticize our neighbor whom we're secretly jealous of. To lash out, in fear of never being good enough.

But what if we were to consider others before ourselves? To exemplify inner confidence by always considering another person's feelings above our own? It certainly wouldn't get ratings on television, but it would result in a more peaceful and harmonious world, a world that advocated love over hate. Isn't this all we want for our children? Unless we can learn the secret to being satisfied with ourselves, our children, our husbands, our belongings, and our careers, the comparisons will never end, and contentment will never start.

FAT TALK

"Oh my gosh! I have gained 10 pounds."

"Are you kidding?! These jeans make me look so fat."

Have you ever verbalized these statements?

Have you ever dieted with a friend or bemoaned the state of your thighs to a workout buddy? Why is it that when we get together with other women, we talk about how much weight we have gained, the latest diet we've tried, or fattening food we shouldn't be eating? Talking with friends about issues related to weight, body dissatisfaction, food, and appearance is not just an everyday occurrence; it's the norm. It is so common psychologists have named it "fat talk." Fat talking is the tendency to make negative comments about our bodies and weight in a social setting. It has become a tried-and-true staple of our feminine culture. Nevertheless, researchers are just beginning to study why we do it and how it affects the way we feel about our bodies and ourselves.

In the early 1990s, anthropologist Mimi Nichter, PhD, unexpectedly stumbled onto "fat talk" while studying teen girls. She noticed during a teen focus group that the girls would engage in a familiar ritual. One girl would say, "I feel so fat," and the other would respond with, "You're not fat!" The exchange was a normal part of daily life; the girls repeated it throughout the day. Once Nichter started listening for fat talk (a term she coined), she realized the ritual was commonplace.

Chances are, you engage in fat talk too. Turning to friends with our concerns is understandable. Relying on friends' support is imperative to healthy functioning. However, do we have to bash our own bodies in order to form this connection? Is it at all healthy for us to do this, not only with each other, but *to* each other and to ourselves? Do we do it for the confirmation that we are *not* actually fat or saggy or out of shape? Or do we really believe what we are saying?

A 2011 study published in the *Psychology of Women Quarterly* found that an "overwhelming majority of women"—93 percent, to be exact—reported having engaged in fat talk. A third of them did it frequently, in association with higher body dissatisfaction and an internalization of a thin ideal.[1]

As a psychologist specializing in eating disorders, Dena has observed firsthand the consequences of negative self-talk, dieting, fat talk, and making disparaging remarks about other people's bodies. Talking about weight and body issues only inspires negative thinking; it creates an atmosphere that perpetuates low esteem and self-loathing. The truth is, most women who engage in fat talk are in a healthy range of their ideal body weight. People who are over their natural weight typically do not engage in fat talk because it hits too close to home. Imagine how a larger person feels when she overhears women in her weight range or lower talking about how fat they feel. It can be very shaming and painful.

Anna Terrey, a private makeup artist who works with women in their late forties and early fifties, listens to fat talk on a daily basis. "Women will say, 'Can you make my face look thinner?', or 'Look at how big my butt looks,' or 'I feel like this blouse is too tight' when it actually looks nice and flattering on her silhouette," she says. "Most of the time, I think women 'fat talk' when they feel insecure and they're not sure how to apply make-up or dress for their bodies."[2]

When Dena sits with her mothers' group and asks how they feel, the answer is most often "fat." In truth, "fat" is a cover-up for sadness or anxiety, but it's easier to say "fat," so Dena validates the feeling then urges, "Tell me what *else* you're feeling," hinting at underlying emotions.

Susan, a mother of one, said she felt "so fat" when she was traveling home on the subway. The heat combined with the close proximity to other passengers increased her body awareness and thus her insecurities. She would then text her best friend about how fat she felt. When she arrived home, she would be so triggered by the negative thoughts and body image struggles that she'd start to binge. After recognizing the negative thought patterns and realizing that the physical discomfort was not about her size but about the crowdedness of the train, Susan began to engage in coping skills—such as leaving on the subway at alternate times and listening to music—instead of venting to her friend.

THE BODY COMPARISON TRAP

Admiring other women while simultaneously criticizing a person's weight, size, or shape is common among most females. We're ambassadors, and tormentors. Advocates, and destroyers.

Women who struggle with disordered eating can be triggered by the attempt to "keep up" with peers in unhealthy ways. We have seen this in numerous cases, some in our own neighborhoods, and some in treatment for serious eating disorders. This is especially true for mothers. How many times have you compared yourself to another mom, thinking, "Why does she appear to have it all together while I am falling apart?" We get caught in the "body comparison trap." We judge ourselves against thinner, more attractive women—a habit that only increases our dissatisfaction with ourselves. It's important to be aware of this tendency and to counter it with a positive response, to focus instead on maintaining healthy, less body-focused relationships with other women.

Dena always tells her children, "Be friends with people that make you feel good about yourself, who are supportive and caring." She tells them to beware of friends who perhaps treat others poorly or who have a negative influence. They may be good people, but not for us. After all, we need to be conscious of our needs and our boundaries. Boundaries are about knowing where someone else ends and we begin.

THE SECRET TO SATISFACTION

The key to being satisfied has nothing to do with what you have, and everything to do with how you have it. It's the Attitude of Gratitude.

How do you hold the gifts God has given you? Your looks, your talents, your belongings, your family? Do you hold them with knuckles white, or do you hold them loosely? Are you willing to share (to let go, even), or are you desperate to cling? Do you foster thankfulness with every bite, with every piece of clean clothing, with every kiss from your daughter, with every embrace from your husband, and do you treasure your wrinkles? Do you treat yourself gently, almost sacredly, being tender with the pulled, the stretched, the tattered parts, knowing you are a gift to so many people?

"As family therapist Peggy Papp reminds us, the quality of a mother's life and her courage are among her most important legacies to her daughter," writes Lerner. "'A woman who can believe in herself when no one else does, who will fight for herself when no one else will, who will continue to struggle even though she is unprotected, this woman demonstrates to her daughter that these possibilities exist.' One great gift a mother can give her daughter is to live her own life as well as possible."[3]

Being a mother is an extremely tall order because we have to become better than ourselves, to live up to the person our child needs us to be. We may be tempted to compare ourselves to the person we *think* our children deserve, but in truth, all we need is to humbly admit what we aren't, and to work on loving who we are. We need to fully embrace the flaws, the brokenness, the inadequacies; to laugh at our clumsy way of living; and to encourage our children to laugh at themselves, too.

"Loving a child doesn't mean giving in to all his whims," said Nadia Boulanger, an internationally renowned music teacher, about the way Leopold Mozart raised Wolfgang. "To love him is to bring out the best in him, to teach him to love what is difficult."[4]

Practice gratitude daily. Make it a habit to praise, to speak positively about yourself when you're looking in the mirror, to turn the negative into a glowing remark, because the spirit in which you treat yourself will, in turn, determine how your children treat themselves.

"In humility, consider others better than yourselves," the Bible tells us (Philippians 2:3). Imagine a world in which people lived this way. In which women praised each other's accomplishments instead of gossiping bitterly. In which people truly wanted what was best for each other.

Emily has always been an introvert. She's not good at small talk, and she shies away from group settings. But when she began fostering two little boys in addition to caring for her own, she soon realized she would need to rely on other people. And so, "Grandma Jo" came on Wednesdays, Angela on Tuesdays, and Miss Carla on Thursdays, to help her dress the boys—all four of them—and to read to them. The kids went swimming with Auntie Karen, fed chickens with Judith, made forts with Juanita, colored with Jen, and played trains with Amber. Other women came in the evenings when Emily's husband was late, helping her bathe the kids and put them to bed, and she even had a friend who folded her laundry.

Because it's women helping women that makes the world grow. Accepting help, and learning to ask for it when you need it, is just as important as helping others. Giving opportunities to others who want to help you is rewarding for them and benefits you and your family. Think about how it makes you feel when you help someone else. Now think about how it would feel if no one ever accepted your help, even to her own detriment and the detriment of her family. Helping reminds us that we are part of a community and that we are surrounded by people who care.

When women get together and refuse to talk badly about each other, it's like a sunrise, all pretty and miraculous. It lights up everything. But when they get together to judge, to gossip, to put down others, it opens a gaping hole in the community into which nothing good can come. If you're a person who engages in such talk, try to stop. And if you're a target, remove yourself from that circle. Nothing positive ever comes from trash-talking our fellow mothers.

EMILY'S STORY

It started when I was nine years old, a homeschooled pastor's kid entering fifth grade. And there were so many skinny girls. It wasn't just that they were skinny. The boys liked them, and here I was in my second-hand clothes and my large plastic glasses, and them chasing me around the playground at recess because of my cheese-and-jam sandwiches.

I hadn't known cheese and jam wasn't "in." I hadn't known I had such fat legs, nor such big glasses, but it was easy for the negative voices to enter because I had no positive ones to counter them. My home was a silent one. There were no compliments or praise, and I didn't think my parents liked me. Whenever I asked if I was beautiful, my mother would remind me that I was being vain, and only inner beauty counted for anything. But all I could see was the outer.

So I stopped bringing cheese and jam to school. Then, I stopped bringing sandwiches to school altogether, in the hopes that one day maybe the boys would like me, too. And I remember one girl in particular. Sabrina Wilson. Tall, blond, slender as a willow branch, she walked as though the world swung on her hips. And the boys followed. She would go on to become a supermodel while I went on to become anorexic.

Later on in high school, after I had begun eating again, I decided that being jealous was a waste of time. Instead, I took what I liked about the girls—perhaps how they dressed or did their hair or walked—and I mimicked them, but there was nothing good in this, either. For I still wasn't being myself. I was just piggybacking on their identities.

Slowly, though, I unearthed myself. And over time, as I began to paint and write and travel, I learned that beauty exists in more shapes than skinny, and in more hair colors than blond. And I began to experiment: I wore a crew cut; I dyed it every color possible, then grew it long and natural and turned it into dreads. I got piercings and tattoos. I no longer compared myself because I'd found myself. And I liked who I found.

Even now, my earlobes are stretched and my hair chopped short. I have two tattoos: one of lilies on my wrist to remind me that I am not much more than grass or flowers—here today and gone tomorrow—but still loved and cared for. And another on my neck, a symbol of the sacred calling of motherhood.

I have little time on this earth. Little time to be me. So why would I spend it being anyone else?

REFLECTION

- When you look at other women, do you automatically compare yourself to them?
- When you look at yourself in the mirror, do you see who you aren't, or do you appreciate who you are?
- Do you talk positively or negatively about your friends behind their backs?
- How do you teach your children to view their classmates and friends?
- What are some ways in which you can inspire love, not jealousy, toward your neighbors, family, and friends?

TOOLS

- Make a list of qualities you love about yourself, and read it over once a day.
- End fat talk.
- Avoid making comments on weight and size, about other people and about yourself.
- Avoid comparing yourself to your friends. If you find yourself comparing, remind yourself of the strengths and gifts you have. Provide positive reassurance.
- If you catch yourself "feeling fat," there may be deeper issues going on. Explore these within yourself.
- When friends tell you they feel fat, don't get into a conversation about weight. Instead, ask how they're doing—dig deeper than the surface.
- If someone makes an unwanted comment about your body, respond with an emphasis on health or character.

- Create a positive relationship with physical exercise. If your friend is a marathon runner, it doesn't mean that you have to be too if you don't even like running. Find something that you enjoy.
- Maintain perspective. As the famous saying goes, "The grass is always greener on the other side."

AS THEY GROW

Your Changing Role
as a Mom and a Woman

Small children disturb your sleep, big children your life.

—Yiddish proverb

WHEN YOUR CHILDREN
TURN TEEN-STRANGERS

You never thought it would happen. You never thought your baby with the pink bows would one day wear a training bra and mascara. You refused to pierce her ears when she was young, and now she has studs lining her lobes and she flashes you angry glances while texting on the cell phone you regretfully bought for her thirteenth birthday. And you rack your brain for what you did wrong, while stuffing Oreos into your mouth to fill the gap that's ever widening between you and your child. The baby who once cooed and laughed and nursed at your breast.

The breast milk has turned sour, so to speak, and your daughter is now threatening to run away unless you let her attend the dance on Friday. You feel torn. You want to put her over your knee, and to cuddle her close. To discipline her, and beg her to forgive you for all the ways you've messed up. Because you love her so much you would die for her but sometimes all you can do is yell, because it's so hard, this parenting. And she is so angry, and all you've ever done is love her.

There are now so many issues to worry about, issues you feel unequipped to deal with: sexuality, boys, drugs, alcohol, and Facebook, and you want to know what she's typing and who she's typing to, and is it wrong to sneak into your child's account when she's asleep to make sure she's safe? You miss the days when you could just hug her and kiss her "owies" and plaster a Dora the Explorer Band-Aid and she would flash you a smile as though you were her superhero. Where are the Band-Aids for a teenager's hurts?

Your son used to tackle your legs and beg you to read him stories, and now he locks himself in his room and plays computer games alone until midnight, or blasts music so loud the walls shake. You want to ask him why, and how he's doing, and to hug away his pain and promise everything will be all right, but he won't even look at you. This is the same boy who used to let you blow kisses on his belly.

So the eating disorder flares up, the one you've managed to ignore for years now, the one your husband never knew you had, and you begin to distract yourself by letting go (of food restraints and appearance), or gripping more tightly (controlling what you eat, exercising more often), because it's easier. Easier than facing the way life is suddenly painful. Or maybe you're someone for whom eating disorders were never a problem, but you're now turning to food for comfort, or overdoing it at the gym to manage the stress.

Lisa had never been overweight, but as her forty-fifth birthday approached, she set out to get in shape. Her sixteen-year-old daughter was running track and Lisa thought it was time that she herself get fit. She started working out in a gym and cutting down on calories and fat. She began taking more walks, and she garnered compliments on her weight loss. But despite Lisa's "healthy" new look, her quest for fitness took a sinister turn.

"The more I exercised and the more I dieted, something just took over me," she recalls. Although she had no prior history of an eating disorder, Lisa's dieting and overexercising spiraled into a full-blown mental illness. This once-fit, healthy, confident mother became severely anorexic, battling body image distortion, low self-esteem, anxiety, depression, and fear of gaining weight. Her life became unmanageable. It's a slippery slope, even as daughters age overnight.

Helen, a close colleague of Dena's, reluctantly admits, "At my age, I long to feel beautiful, thin, and energetic. I am envious of my seventeen-year-old daughter. I hate that she is prettier, smaller, and thinner than me. It makes me miss my youth and despise my age."

You were embarrassed of your mother, and now your children are embarrassed of you. You used to take your daughter on shopping sprees and she would confide in you. Now she scowls at you as though there's lipstick on your teeth, so you diet and binge and spend hours at the gym. As the Italian proverb goes, "Little children, headache; big children, heartache."

Dr. Kathryn Zerbe, a professor of psychiatry at Oregon Health and Science University and the author of *The Body Betrayed: A Deeper Understanding of Women, Eating Disorders and Treatment*, asserts that older women must be able to mourn in order to adjust to life-altering events such as the loss of youthful appearance and changes in relationships.[1] While mourning, however, it's important to remember, *this too shall pass*. The teenage years—while long—do not last forever. Family therapist and author Virginia Satir said in *The New Peoplemaking*, "Adolescents are not monsters. They are just people trying to learn how to make it among the adults in the world, who are probably not so sure themselves."[2]

HOW TO LOVE ON OLDER CHILDREN

Parents of toddlers and teens can attest to the fact that true love often doesn't feel like love at all. Rather, it feels like gut-wrenching agony. It would seem that teenagers are just another version of toddlers—only older. They both whine, and throw tantrums, and feel sorry for themselves when really, the whole world caters to them. Judith Martin, author of *Miss Manners' Guide to Rearing Perfect Children*, said, "The invention of the teenager was a mistake. Once you identify a period of life in which people get to stay out late but don't have to pay taxes—naturally, no one wants to live any other way."[3]

But there are ways to love on teenagers that don't necessarily spoil them. Ways to communicate that will bridge the gap, but this requires learning their language. The language of the teen is nonverbal. It listens, it holds, it watches, it prays. It lets go of, and trusts and weeps and waits. It provides flowers and freshly folded laundry and kisses at night, even when those kisses are unwanted. It is consistent and patient; it writes notes, slid beneath doors; and it does not judge or give up or put down.

Start When They're Young

Waiting until the teenage years to communicate is like trying to run a marathon without ever having trained. Spend your life learning your children—their favorite color, favorite dessert, favorite band. According to Gary Chapman and Ross Campbell, authors of *The Five Love Languages of Children*, five techniques exist for learning your child's "love languages" (Physical Touch, Gifts, Words of Affirmation, Quality Time, and Acts of Service) in our sons and daughters.

1. Observe how your child expresses love to you.

"Watch your child," write Chapman and Campbell. "He may well be speaking his own language. This is particularly true of a young child, who is very likely to express love to you in the language he desires most to receive."

Emily's two-year-old is one of the most caring people she knows. When his brother is crying, she often doesn't get there in time, Aiden having already run across the room to pat Kasher's tummy and bring him toy after toy. While it's still too early to know for sure, it would seem that one of Aiden's predominant love languages is Acts of Service.

Her foster child, however, could spend an hour snuggled up to someone. His primary love language is therefore Physical Touch.

2. Observe how your child expresses love to others.

Perhaps your daughter spends hours making or purchasing presents for people, not just at Christmastime, but throughout the year. This would imply that her way of expressing love is through Gifts.

3. Listen to what your child requests most often.

If your child frequently desires to know how she looks, or what you think of her artwork, it's most likely her love language is Words of Affirmation.

4. Notice what your child most frequently complains about.

If your daughter says things like, "You never have time for me," or "Why won't you play house with me?" this is indicative that her love language is Quality Time.

5. Give your child a choice between two options.

"As you give options for several weeks, keep a record of your child's choices," write Campbell and Chapman. "If most of them tend to cluster around one of the five love languages, you have likely discovered which one makes your child feel most loved. At times, your child will not want either option, and will suggest something else. You should keep a record of those requests also, since they may give you clues."[4]

When she becomes a teenager, however, your child's love languages—no matter how well known or fulfilled—will fluctuate. "Because of the changes they are experiencing, your teens' giving and receiving of love may also change with their moods," warn Chapman and Campbell.[5] Just remain cool, calm, and pleasant as your children flounder around gasping for air and testing your faithfulness to them. Leave your bedroom door open so they can talk to you. Be accepting while firm, and let them know they are safe with you. Make time for them. Never make them feel unwanted—even when they are.

Baker tells this story: "It's late. Only nine p.m. But so late. The night shift will soon begin and the day shift with bath-times and teeth brushing battles has only just begun to wind down. I slink away for a bit to steal some quiet and maybe some few moments of sleep in between shifts.

"But . . . he's clambering in and behind me, pulling the blankets, readjusting the pillows, talking all the while.

"'Mama, can we chat?'

"I force myself to think very slowly. To process the words before they come out of my mouth so that what he hears isn't, 'No, no, no please leave me alone before Zoe wakes up again' but instead, 'Yes, I'd love to chat with you, Jackson. *I love you.*'

"That's what I need him to hear. With his ears and his heart. So we snuggle in the warm dark and he talks. . . . And he pauses now and again to exclaim as if in surprise how much he loves me and I repeat it back and we both revel in the reconnecting. The rediscovering that we actually like each other as much as we love each other."[6]

So, friends, let's pull back the covers of our hearts, and let's welcome our children in. Before it's too late.

Don't Take It Personally

It's not easy. After giving your time, energy, and life to this tiny person, you're suddenly being treated like you don't exist—or worse, like your existence is repulsive. Any person, no matter how strong her self-esteem, would be in pain. You have a right to feel hurt. You do. But don't cry about it to your children; don't nag and complain. That will only push them further away.

Instead, vent to your husband or to your friends. Take strength from the fact that you are not alone: mothers (and fathers) everywhere are underappreciated, underloved, and overwhelmed by their teenage children. Lerner says this: "Almost all daughters (and sons) feel disappointed with their mothers at some point, because nobody can live up to the impossible and exhausting expectations that accompany mothering. Your daughter's mistake will probably be to assume that she's going to get it 'right' when she becomes a mother herself, rather than questioning gender roles and the job description itself.

"Your daughter may blast you somewhere along the way, especially if she's confident that you're sturdy enough to take it. Mothers are less apt to disappear in the fray than fathers, so you may well get blamed for the behavior of two.

"Expect your daughter to be upset, not only with your imperfect mothering, but also because you didn't see options to live your life or conduct your relationships differently. Some of your daughter's complaints will be true, since you can't possibly get it right all—or even much—of the time. Sometimes it is only after we are able to hear our daughter's criticisms and anger, and are open to apologizing for the inevitable hurts and mistakes that every parent makes, that we can expect to be truly heard by our daughters. Try to be a good listener."[7]

It is easier to withstand a teenager's coldness when you realize that it is not necessarily reflective of your parenting, but instead, reflective of the child-turning-teenager-turning-adult angst. A metamorphosis of sorts. Your child is growing and stretching and needing somehow to separate herself from you, to distinguish herself from you, in order to become who she needs to be, and this hurts. So when you are trying to bridge the gap and are met with stony glances or bedroom doors, don't turn to the fridge. Remember to be kind, because as Plato says, all of us are fighting a battle.[8]

The teenage years are a growth spurt of mammoth proportion, and every period of growth includes feeding and hibernation. Feeding off friends and music and art and computer games, and hibernating in silence, away from those whom know you best. But also *actual* feeding (how many moms of teenagers lament their frequent trips to the grocery store?) And sleeping—some teenagers will sleep through entire days when they can. Recognizing that their bodies need nourishment and rest and helping them to get both in healthy doses will help to smooth out some of the rough.

Let Them Go

It's similar to deciding what one believes; you can't ride the coattails of your parents to church your whole life. Well, you could, but you would look pretty ridiculous, so at some point, your child needs to let go and learn to walk on his own. Like any developmental stage, adolescence is one step further in independence, and something you, as a mother, both want and resist. After all, your child feels like your personal possession. Like he or she belongs to you. When you have this idea in mind, it's easy to become bitter when your baby begins to pull away.

Again, it's all about perspective. About the gratitude attitude, about seeing this daughter or son as a gift, and remembering that gifts are just that. Our children belong to the One who made them—the Creator—and not to us. Nevertheless, as much as we spiritualize and compartmentalize and philosophize about the teen years, there is no denying that they're tough. "Of all the counseling I've done and from my reading I can say . . . oh, my, age 13 can be a hard year," said counselor and author Jean Lush on the Focus on the Family program *Mothers and Sons*. "I'll give you an example from our family. This mother noticed her son was in a bad mood and she said, 'Oh, do come over and see these photographs and help me choose which one I'll use for Christmas. They're photos of myself.'

"The boy came over and said, 'I don't like any of them. Your breath stinks. I'm going to my room.' The mother said, 'Oh, I was so hurt.' But two hours later the boy came out and said, 'I love you, Mom.'

"A little boy achieves male maturity over his mother's dead body. . . . He doesn't just kill her; he 'stabs' her slowly.

"Let me explain. I think many little boys are afraid of the male thing ahead. Not all of them are like this of course. Some just sail through, but there are others that ask anxiously, 'Will I ever become a proper male?' In those cases, the mother is in his way. If she is too close, the child may feel swallowed up by her. After all, she is a woman. She stands between him and being a man. The boys who struggle most are sometimes the ones who have had the closest relationship with their mothers.

"So what do they have to do to get her out of the way? They have to 'kill' her. Killing is the little boy who said, 'Your breath stinks.' This was his way of establishing his masculinity. That episode was very hard for the mother, who felt rejected and wounded by her son, but it was a transition they had to endure.

"Mothers whose sons suddenly go through this kind of alienation are inclined to ask themselves, 'What am I doing wrong? I don't know what to do. The kid is a little tyrant.' Well, hang in there. Better days are coming."[9]

Consider the Heavens

During this time of extreme testing, be good to yourself. To the extent possible, do not take out your anxiety on food or work or exercise, but instead, turn to something larger and recognize what it might be asking of you. Keep your door ajar and make an effort to truly see your children. Open your eyes wide and observe when they need a hug, when they need time alone, when they are hungry or tired or lonely. And don't preach. Just open your arms and your ears, and listen. Even when it hurts, and even when they're telling you things you don't want to hear, just listen.

Up until now, you've spent so many years teaching right from wrong that it's time to trust. We realize you can't trust your children completely, but you can try—and believe it or not, they will want to honor you for trying. At the end of the day, despite our best efforts, not all children will turn out the way we want or the way we expect. It's okay to accept that this is the way it is. To accept that we don't have control over everything, even over how our children turn out. And in those instances it's okay to say you had no control, that you did the best you could.

Andrew was the first of four children born into an upper-middle-class family. He played sports growing up with his father as coach, took family vacations, and spent time with his parents and his grandparents. When he wasn't doing well in school, Andrew had tutors. He went to church regularly and took the sacraments. His mother stayed home to tend to the family until the youngest was in full-day grade school; all six of them ate dinner together every night. They lived in a good community with strong families. In his later high-school years and early twenties, Andrew got hooked on drugs and began dealing them locally. He failed college, and he had fights and run-ins with the law. He couldn't hold a job. His parents stood by him, doing whatever they could to help him. After several attempts to move out and start a life of his own, he could not break the cycle of addiction. Nearly ten years later, he met and earned the love of a good woman and they settled down; he attended AA and straightened out most of his problems. He works a modest job now and has two children, but it was a long and painful road.

At the same time, the other three children excelled in school, went on to college, had no troubles with drugs or alcohol or legal scrapes, found good jobs, married, settled down, and had children. They were well behaved and well liked throughout their childhoods and young adult years. What made one child have such a difficult time? They all had the same parents, the same opportunities, and the same support system, yet only one had issues so monumental that they threatened to take his life. In the end, no amount of love and guidance could help Andrew. He had to find his own way and to sort things out for himself. Despite the pain his parents endured watching him during this time, they were essentially powerless once he reached a certain age.

And sometimes we're all powerless, and we have to accept that. We don't have to stand by and watch our children sink—we can throw them a lifeline—but it's up to them to grab hold of it. Nevertheless, there is hope. Often the greatest lessons have the highest cost, but so long as there is life, there is hope. Trust that Someone Bigger is watching out for your child. This is not the end.

EMILY'S STORY

For two years during my anorexia, I didn't let my parents hug me. It was my way of punishing them for not being who I needed them to be. But sometimes at night, I'd hear Mum sneaking into my room when she thought I was sleeping, and she'd lie down beside me just so she could hold me. And it felt good.

But I didn't let her know this. I couldn't let her know because then I might stop being angry, and the anger fueled my eating disorder and made me skinny. So I kept being angry. Angry at them for not hugging me more, even though I wouldn't let them. Angry at them for raising me like a geek, when the world told me I should be cool. Angry that I wasn't more beautiful, angry that I was so lonely, angry that life was often heartache. And it was a twisted circle, like the vine of a sweet pea that had lost its blooms.

I wanted my mother to enter into the hard places with me. To sit on my bed, where I measured my wrists every day after school and sobbed. I wanted her to hear me. But I think she was afraid of what I might say. Because no daughter of hers would ever get an eating disorder. She had decided this when we were young, when she wouldn't let us play with Barbies. This is the danger of having too-high of expectations for our children, of weighing them down with our fears.

My mother's hugging me at night was a touch that told me I mattered, and I think, for children, this *is* what matters: to know they are important to someone, to know they are worth running down the prodigal laneway to kiss and clothe and feast with, despite their spending the family inheritance. And today, I believe I matter in the way of leaving my hands in the dishwater for five minutes, just to feel them soften, and the heat becomes a spa becomes a mother's mini-paradise. "This is heaven," I tell Trenton, holding a hot washcloth to my face, and he laughs. "You're easy to please," he says, and again and always, it's about perspective. Seeing the washcloth for what it could be.

I believe I matter in the slow light of winter, hearing the crunch of boot and the call of the cardinal and refusing to hurry the holy. I believe I matter in the baring of husband's skin, in the placing of hand on the seed that grows within me, in the laughing out loud, so loud, in the middle of the grocery store. For we do. We matter. Enough for our Creator to kneel toward earth, blow dust into swirls into DNA, and pat us perfect in the Garden of Eden. And if we believe this hard enough, eventually maybe our children will, too.

REFLECTION

- How has your role as a mother changed and developed as your children have grown?
- How has your self-esteem altered since your son or daughter became a teenager? Why do you think this is?
- Did you take the time to listen to your kids when they were young? Did you truly see them?

- What about your relationship with your children would you like to change now, if you could?
- How has being a teenager turned your child into a stranger?

TOOLS

- Even if you didn't pay attention to your children when they were young, it's never too late. Start now. Plan an outing or just visit their bedroom; whatever you do, come in peace. Bring flowers, or a bag of chips, or something that acts as an offering, and even if it doesn't go over well the first time, try and try again. Perseverance develops character, and character, hope.
- Write a letter to your teenager, telling her how much she means to you and asking forgiveness for the ways in which you've inadvertently, or purposely, hurt her in the past.
- Allow as much freedom as possible without compromising your beliefs; let your child play her music in the living room so she doesn't have to stay closed up in her room all the time. Let her bring her boyfriend to supper; invite her life into yours. And remember: the teenage years are temporary. Love and life are eternal.
- Go through photos of yourself from the past decade. Describe what you think or feel when you look at each picture. Consider how you viewed your body in each photo. What was your awareness or self-image at the time of the picture? What stages were your personal growth and development at? How does that compare to now? What part does aging play in the years of negative body image? If your body looks the same, address the similarities or differences in how you felt or feel. Do your life experiences enable you to have a different view of your body now?

GETTING HELP

Hope and a Cure

Eating is not a crime. It's not a moral issue. It's normal. It's enjoyable. It just is.

—Carrie Arnold

IS COMPLETE HEALING POSSIBLE?

We all need healing. Whether we're overweight or underweight or average, whether we're old or young or in between, our image of the body has been broken and needs fixing. Healing takes on different forms. For some of us who have battled severe eating disorders—the clinical kind, such as anorexia nervosa, bulimia nervosa, or binge eating disorder—it means rehabilitation until we are strong enough mentally to make positive choices for our lives. We may want to get better. We may choose to get better. But it requires months of treatment and years of reorienting one's mind-set to truly recover.

For others of us, who struggle with body image but have never experienced a clinical disorder, it's about choosing healing on a daily, more ordinary basis. It's about choosing to love ourselves enough to eat healthfully. It's about choosing to accept our bodies as they are. Choosing to believe we are worth the food on our plates and the reflection in the mirror. Choosing to get regular exercise. These choices require discipline as well as tools we can employ when we're not up to caring for ourselves, and the motivation for becoming comfortable in our own skin.

It sounds easy, right? Like you just make a choice and it happens. Not necessarily. If you struggle with a diagnosed eating disorder, body image issues, disturbance with food, low self-esteem, or any other issues that cause you to feel repulsed or sad when you look in the mirror, it is not your fault. These issues stem from transgenerational, genetic, socio-cultural, and gender issues that are global and complex. Researchers and experts in the field explain that some people inherit a brain chemistry that makes them more prone to food problems, thus putting them more at risk for body image issues. Also, there is a genetic link between eating disorders, anxiety, and depression. The picture is complicated and illus-trates the fact that there is not one cause or reason for the difficulties with food issue or body image disturbance.

However, you alone must take responsibility for healing. And that starts with insight, awareness, and then the choice to improve your life by taking steps to do so. That is what this book is about—helping you to overcome the barriers that interfere with your quality of life, and to acquire the tools and skills that will allow you to make the choice to recover.

Sometimes you have to choose every single day, or sometimes ev-ery minute, to accept and change. When Dena was a young adult she was in a car accident that was not her fault, but every day she had to choose to get out of bed and rehabilitate. She was not alone and had a tremendous amount of support, but ultimately it was up to her to make the decision to get better.

Our minds have been sabotaged. They've gone through an incred-ible ordeal during and after pregnancy, and are so busy catching up from years of abuse that they've forgotten, in some ways, how to func-tion normally. Give it time. Be kind to yourself—treat yourself like a trauma victim—and minister to the wounded places. In the meantime, trust the people God has put in your life. The team of professionals who can guide you back to health.

THE TEN PHASES OF RECOVERY

Carolyn Costin, a recovered disordered eater and founder of the Monte Nido Treatment Center in Malibu, California, believes that healing consists of ten phases (or *phrases*):

1. I don't think I have a problem.
2. I might have a problem, but it's not that bad.
3. I have a problem, but I don't care.
4. I want to change, but I don't know how, and I'm scared.
5. I tried to change, but I couldn't.
6. I can stop some of the behaviors, but not all of them.
7. I can stop the behaviors but not my thoughts.
8. I am often free from behaviors, and thoughts, but not all the time.
9. I am free from behaviors and thoughts.
10. I am recovered.[1]

"Being recovered is when a person can accept his or her natural body size and shape and no longer has a self-destructive relationship with food or exercise," Costin explains. "When you are recovered, food and weight take a proper perspective in your life, and what you weigh is not more important than who you are; in fact, actual numbers are of little or no importance at all.

"When recovered, you will not compromise your health or betray your soul to look a certain way, wear a certain size, or reach a certain number on a scale. When you are recovered you do not use eating disorder behaviors to deal with, distract from, or cope with other problems."[2]

As a society, we tend to want quick fixes, but there is no quick fix to disordered eating or poor body image. It is a long journey, and relapses are unfortunately inevitable. There is no set cause for an eating disorder, and therefore no particular cure, but the good news is that with true healing—a holistic kind of healing—comes freedom: of mind, soul, and body.

Emily has told her story of anorexia a few times on a Christian daily talk show. The one thing she finds hard is the host's insistence on her being cured of anorexia. In some sense of the word, we do believe full healing is possible. It is possible, with time, to retrain the mind to think positive and lovely thoughts about oneself; to retrain the body to trust its hunger cues; to retrain the heart to trust in God, or in whatever or whoever has hurt it. But it all takes time. And just because healing happens doesn't mean a person can't get sick again. This is why it's important for us to know our triggers. To know them, so we can stay away from them.

It's important to take preventative measures to keep your life in balance. Try to be proactive instead of reactive. A balanced lifestyle is critical for keeping life stressors, world pressures, and the daily grind in check. Priorities need to be constantly evaluated and relationships and connections, nourished.

Body image issues may never totally dissipate. We will still have days when we look in the mirror and fight with our mother, days filled with piles of laundry and pressures at work. Days in which we take out our stress on our loved ones and our bodies. But we can grow, in spite of it all. We can become aware of these moments, and then step back and try to figure out what is really going on. When we start to do this, our bodies become less of a target and we discover the real source of what we are feeling. And when we look in the mirror and don't like what we see, we can begin to ask, "How am I out of balance? What do I need to change in my life?'"

For Emily, these triggers include the nutrition graphs on food packages, or anything to do with calories, diets, or weigh scales. Like a former alcoholic avoiding the bar, or liquor stores, or alcoholics, Emily has to steer clear of these obstacles or potential setbacks. This doesn't mean she isn't healed. It just means she's human and has to continue to take care of herself even after returning to a healthy threshold. We aren't invincible. And it would be foolish to assume that the thing that happened once can't happen again. We are wiser for the fall, but shouldn't return to the very path that caused us to stumble.

ARM YOURSELF

That being said, it is important to walk in the hope of one day being healed. To rise from bed each morning speaking positive words to your reflection; to see loveliness in the mirror, not shame. To acknowledge that you feel sad, and that this is okay, and that your feelings don't determine your value as a person.

"This is a call to arms," writes Valerie Monroe. "A call to be gentle, to be forgiving, to be generous with yourself. The next time you look into the mirror, try to let go of the story line that says you're too fat or too sallow, too ashy or too old, your eyes are too small or your nose too big; just look into the mirror and see your face. When the criticism drops away, what you will see then is just you, without judgment, and that is the first step toward transforming your experience of the world."[3]

It is also important to surround yourself with accountability partners, with people who adore you, who aren't afraid to speak the truth in love. People whom you call, bawling, saying you've done it again: you've eaten five Mars bars and a chocolate cake and it still didn't fill the hole. People who remind you that tomorrow is a new day, and that you are a new creation.

In addition to having accountability, you need to know your hangups. Perhaps it's flipping through fashion magazines, weighing yourself, or being around people who talk about food. Perhaps it is stress regarding your job or your children that sets you off. Maybe it's arguing with your spouse or your parents. Recognizing and acknowledging these triggers is a start toward knowing yourself and understanding that the disordered eating is not about food. It's about the situation surrounding the food. Realizing this is the first step toward healing; it opens your eyes and gives you control over your circumstances and how you respond.

RECOVERY VERSUS CURE

Recovery versus Cure is a topic of incredible dissension and conflict in the eating disorders field. Professionals argue about whether one can truly be cured, or if one is always in recovery. Another source of division is considering what constitutes recovery. What really matters, however, is not if you call yourself "cured" or "recovered/recovering," but whether or not these words have any meaning. We do know, without a doubt, that recovery or healing or whatever you want to call it is absolutely possible. Not only has Emily gone through it herself, but we have spoken to countless women and girls who have experienced freedom from their eating disorder. They have claimed, promised, and declared that an eating disorder sufferer can be healed.

In our opinion, being recovered means you have finally let yourself become a real, connected human being. You have found a purpose beyond your appearance; your identity is not connected to food, weight, size, or shape. Recovery is about having the courage to express emotions and deal with stress. It is about freedom from food and its dominion over life and issues. It is about spiritual connection. It is about improving friendships and relationships with significant others. Ultimately, freedom constitutes a better life.

As one of Dena's patients, who's been recovered for four years, put it, "Recovery is . . . a journey, different for all who embark upon it. Recovery enables you to gain confidence as you grow out of a life-threatening disease and addiction. Recovery is not about an individual's status. It is a journey of the heart, fighting against lies that want nothing more than to destroy the very reason any person exists. Recovery is a choice. Though it is not easy, for those like myself who want nothing more than to say, 'I am living recovered,' it is a choice that must be made."

Another former sufferer shared a somewhat different perspective: "We girls in recovery want to hear . . . hopeful future versions of ourselves. They are like long-lost family members that, after emigrating to a new country, never wrote back to their families . . . to tell how lovely their new homes were. We never heard back from them. . . .

"So this is my letter back home. This is my letter to my brothers and sisters who want to know what this mystical land of Recovery looks like. It's great. I'm free. It's frighteningly, incredibly, undeniably possible, this priceless freedom of Recovery."

BELIEVE IN SOMETHING GREATER

The hardest part about letting go of disordered eating is that for a while, you lose yourself. You don't know who you are anymore. Disordered eating gives you a sense of identity—one that makes you feel more in control than being a wife or a mother ever will.

But the ED identity is a lie. As author Lisa Bevere writes, "It has grown from a seed, a word, a disapproving glance, a rejection, a comparison. It was planted deep into the soil of a wound in your soul during a time (or many times) when rejection or acceptance of you as a person was based on your physical form. Or perhaps it was planted during a time when your person was violated in such a painful way that you decided to barricade your *self* physically from the world, rather than endure that kind of pain again. Or perhaps you just bowed under the weight of the constant barrage of negative, accusing messages sent by our cultural advertising and negligent entertainment media.

"How can one resist and overcome such influences? How can wounds so deep and secret ever be healed? You must first *know who you really are*. As a human, you are created in the image of God, and there are multiple dimensions of you."[4]

We are not our appearance. We are multifaceted, and were put on earth to reflect something greater than ourselves: to emanate goodness, love, kindness, joy, and peace. However, we can learn to believe in something greater only by losing focus of ourselves. We need to look past the reflection in the mirror and find the purpose beyond that reflection. We can live fully only when we live selflessly. We rob ourselves when we speak unkindly or think critical thoughts about ourselves or our neighbors. Just as food distracts a disordered eater, hate and judgment distract us from fulfilling a purpose that was determined for us before we were born. We can change the world, but it's all about love. Until we learn to love our very existence, to believe we are worth something simply because we live and breathe and move, until we learn to show grace to ourselves and to embrace the house—the body—in which we live, and to treat it kindly, we will be unable to reflect anything greater.

STOP LIVING IN THE PAST

Walking in our true, multifaceted identity requires letting go of the past. It requires acknowledging our hurt, and then releasing it. Food often becomes a vacuum that sucks up all the sadness. Except there are always more tears, and so, more food, and it's a way of obsessing to forget. To forget the way we have no control over people's getting older, over our parents' needing care, over our children's getting sick, over our friends' dying or moving away or deciding suddenly not to be friendly anymore. And you hear that heaven is real and God is love and Jesus came to save you, but the church is the coldest place you've ever visited and the pew makes your back hurt. So why would you turn to faith when you could open up a bag of chips?

The hardest thing in the world is often to do nothing. To stop trying, and to simply sit in sadness and acknowledge it. To see the sadness for what it is, to embrace it, and to accept that the world is not as it should be. Unless we do this, we cannot fully be saved because we won't realize we need saving. We'll be too busy trying to forget, and by the time we remember, it will be too late, so put down the sandwich and let yourself feel. Then release it all, put it behind you, and leave it there.

We can put the past behind us, though, only by forgiving ourselves, and then accepting the pain that has been afflicted on us. So first, we let ourselves feel the pain. We acknowledge the bruises, and we mourn them. But then, we accept. Acceptance does not mean that you condone what has happened to you, nor does it mean that the person or the event warrants it. No, we accept because to accept is to set ourselves free from bitterness. Acceptance often leads to forgiveness. And this can be the next step in the healing process. We forgive because we, too, make mistakes, and we, too, need forgiveness. God accepts us as we are and in turn, has offered us his forgiveness, so we, in turn, need to do the same to others.

And forgiveness isn't easy. It's not a feeling, either. It's a decision. One very similar to deciding to love yourself. You tell yourself every day that you're beautiful. And you tell yourself every day that you forgive the other person. And over time (similar to pretending to like someone who gets on your nerves) this action will feel more natural. And you will become free of your clutch on the past. Free to embrace the future.

TREATMENT GUIDELINES

NEDA's Perspective

If you struggle with disordered eating or know of someone who does, the National Eating Disorders Association (NEDA) emphasizes the importance of getting help at the appropriate level of care that corresponds to the severity of your eating disorder. "There are goals and markers to determine the right level of care," states the *NEDA Navigator Guidebook*. "The American Psychiatric Association (APA)[5] publishes practice guidelines that are very accessible and readable online."[6]

Eating disorder professionals are familiar with this guide and will use it to help determine the level of care that is best for you. NEDA believes that it's important to have a team of professionals involved, including a physician to address the medical issues; a psychiatrist to handle medication; a nutritionist to work on dietary concerns; and a clinician/psychologist to undertake individual, family, or group therapy.

"You might try thinking about this disorder in the same way that would be applied to an individual suffering from a brain injury," the guidebook says. "Just like the brain-injured patient, the ED patient needs a team of specialists to address the multifarious issues associated with the illness, and each patient is unique in how the illness manifests or 'shows up. . . .'" A specialist team is perhaps particularly important for anorexics, for another reason: anorexics sometimes have difficulty connecting with others. They should be exposed to multiple caregivers so the chances of them connecting with at least one are higher.

"For example, an anorexic may hear the same information from four different caregivers, but the information doesn't register or 'click' until the fifth caregiver says it."[7]

In other words, it's important to have help along the way, and to continue seeking that help. If you do not suffer from an actual eating disorder, but you still have poor self-esteem, getting counseling is a wise option. Talking to a professional can open up a new field of vision for you, helping you to make peace with your body and with yourself.

Our Perspective

Having worked in the field for more than two decades, Dena believes that treatment centers and providers are not created equal. Treatment has changed dramatically over the past ten years, particularly in the United States, where managed care has gotten a foothold. It is therefore important when seeking treatment to research fully, both the facility and its employees. In addition, get recommendations; talk to the alumni and ask questions. For example, is the organization Joint Commission accredited (a standard of care for mental health facilities)? If it's an individual rather than a facility, is the individual licensed? Pay attention to the facility's website; is it updated regularly, or does it remain stagnant? Does the institution itself attract you, or is it sterile and cold? Is the organization itself clinically or insurance driven? Does it value the continuity of care? Does it use evidence-based treatment and offer a comprehensive multimodal approach (integrating biopsychosocial models of recovery as well as best practices including client views)? Furthermore, do employees display compassion, respect, and experience?

From a spiritual standpoint, we would argue that while all treatment facilities are valuable, only some address the needs of the soul—the underlying issues that feed the root of the problem in the first place. In choosing treatment, it is therefore important to consider whether or not one's faith is of importance, and if it is, to opt for a faith-based facility that will tenderly address the spiritual side of things, as well as the physical, mental, and emotional.

Timely intervention is of the utmost importance. Evidence-based and best practices delivered by qualified and experienced health professionals, including medical, nutritional, psychological, and psychopharmacologic services is mandatory. Family involvement should be a priority in treatment whenever possible.

A multidisciplinary approach is imperative and reflects the complex issues encompassing an eating disorder. An eating disorder is a culmination of biological, psychological, social, and spiritual issues. Thus, an interdisciplinary team is necessary to address all these dimensions of an eating disorder. Furthermore, treatment approaches should include cognitive behavioral therapy, dialectical behavior therapy, and motivational approaches.

Levels of care range from the most restrictive environment including inpatient and residential care, in which the patient resides at the facility, to intensive outpatient day programs and outpatient treatment in which the patient lives at home. Inpatient programs allow for a patient to be given twenty-four-hour care at a live-in facility. Psychiatric and physical health assistance are included, and patients tend to stay at treatment facilities for months at a time. Various assessments determine a patient's acceptance into this high-maintenance treatment. A crucial difference between inpatient and outpatient care is the amount of medical attention received by a patient. Inpatient care includes constant supervision, monitoring of positive or negative health levels, and emergency care if a person's health is declining. Overall, it tends to be more intensive due to its structured and defined atmosphere. It helps the individual forget about life's distractions and focuses instead on physical and psychological healing. In contrast, outpatient treatment does not generally address medical conditions or nutritional needs. It is desirable largely because of its flexibility. Adults with children who cannot afford months of treatment find it to be a very positive alternative.

Questions to consider when deciding between the two include:

- **How much can you afford to spend?** Overall, outpatient treatment is cheaper because housing is not included and fewer hours of treatment and therapy are offered.
- **Are you willing to put in the extra work required of outpatient treatment?** Without constant supervision, it is easier for eating disorder patients to give in to temptation, particularly during the early stages of treatment.
- **If you attend inpatient treatment, what support will you be given when you leave?** When making your choice, it is important to consider the kind of follow-up care provided by an inpatient facility.

- **Is your condition severe?** If the answer is yes, inpatient care may be necessary. If the problem is finances, many facilities offer grants and scholarships. Don't be afraid to call the institution in question and query about financial aid so that money doesn't stand between you and recovery.

EMILY'S STORY

I walk the halls of the eating disorder clinic in Edmonton, Alberta, biting my lip to keep from crying over the girls lining the floor on mattresses and blankets, these shrunken frames, emaciated faces, and eyes as empty as the walls. It's an anorexic holocaust.

"Why are they lying on the ground?" I ask the girl I've come to visit, a girl whose mother has written me begging for help.

"They're the outpatients," she says. "They don't have rooms, so they bring their own beds."

She's a Christian girl, with blond hair and blue eyes, and she's nearly all bone. And even though I find these bones repulsive now, I have to be careful when I enter these places because the sickness is infectious. And I can't listen to these girls talking about calories or food because then I remember. I remember what it's like to think that way.

I go to the clinic occasionally, when a parent begs me to, but otherwise I prefer just to visit the families. It's hard to be faced with a disorder that used to be mine. It's not something I am proud of. I wish I could forget it, but I can't, particularly since I relapsed as a young married woman and put my husband through it too. And I didn't get professional treatment either time.

At age thirteen, I was admitted into a general hospital where they handed me a tray full of food and told me to eat or they'd feed me intravenously. Thankfully, I was ready to get better, after four years of starving and nearly dying and the nurses calling me a miracle. The second time, at twenty-six, I didn't get treatment either—even though now I wish I had. I simply began eating again after my husband gave me an ultimatum, telling me I needed to choose between him and food. But this time, I knew healing would take more than downloading menus from the Internet. Because I'd relapsed, I knew that it wasn't just a case of "to eat or not to eat." I'd never really sat down and analyzed why I wasn't eating. All I knew was that I felt better, calmer, safer, and more attractive when I was hungry. As though I'd become part of some noble cause.

I am still figuring out the reasons for this disorder, and it's been five years since I last recovered. The more you starve yourself, the more confused your brain becomes and the less rational your decisions—such as mine, to drink multiple cups of coffee each day so I wouldn't feel the hunger, not realizing that coffee was causing my insomnia. I had so many hurts, so many disappointments stuffed inside of me that it took years for them to resurface, and when they did, on my wedding day, I hurriedly shoved them back down.

We don't know how to handle our emotions. We name them wrong and don't take the time to get to know them. By sitting in the broken place, however, we allow ourselves to become acquainted with the hard pit of bitterness; with the gray ash that is sadness; with the yellow light that is joy. By giving our feelings a name and a shape, we validate them, and in turn, we validate ourselves.

REFLECTION

- Do you like the person you've become over the years? Why or why not?
- Do you feel as though disordered eating, or the diet mentality, has taken over your life?
- Do you want help?
- Do you believe there is freedom and hope beyond the bondage to food?
- What has prevented you from getting treatment, or seeing a counselor, prior to now?
- At what point, if any, do you think you'd be ready to seek help?

TOOLS

- Ask your husband and children whether or not they think you need help when it comes to your relationship with food and with yourself.

- Research the institutions, clinics, and rehabs available, and consider whether or not you could benefit from their programs.
- Book an appointment with a psychologist or therapist and get a professional's opinion.

IDENTITY CRISIS

Discovering True Self-Worth

This is what we do, my mother's life said. We find ourselves in the sacrifices we make.

—Cammie McGovern

THE WAY WE SEE

Perhaps we have it backward. Maybe it's not about size at all, but about strength. Maybe it's not about smooth skin, but about wrinkles. Maybe instead of coloring our roots, it's about showing off our silver hairs. Maybe it's all about perspective.

When a person looks at an oak tree, he sees strength—not size. When he cuts down this tree, he doesn't airbrush the rings, but marvels at their number. Like wrinkles, they display age and long suffering, tales untold. So why do we try to cover up our stories? Society has chosen certain qualifiers like size, smoothness of skin, and color of hair because it can profit from them. It cannot profit from natural, God-given beauty. It cannot market true value. So, using commercials and movies and sitcoms, it saturates our brains with the need to appear fake so it can turn a nice dollar. It trains us to feel inadequate, watching the young, shapely, fit women in commercials and "reality shows," and we start to despise ourselves. We become like children with toy ads, and it doesn't matter how many toys we already have. All we can think is, *I need more*. Because society tells us we do. The cycle spirals, and we get work done on our noses, boobs, eyebrows, thighs, and lips, until we're so plastic we can no longer smile. Because we've lost the sense of what it means to be real, to have the marks on our bodies telling the story of our lives.

North American media have hit the world with Barbie bombshells. They have destroyed the lives and souls of hundreds of thousands of girls, all in the name of profit. Even women who do not experience eating disorders find themselves tied up in knots over not looking like the trophy wife some hotshot Hollywood executive parades around for movie premieres—and just look at her abs, just three months after she had twins!

In the beginning, it seemed simple enough. Eat a little less, get a little thinner. Dye your hair, and feel a bit better about yourself. But soon it escalated into counting calories and exercising for hours and spending money you didn't have, all because you didn't measure up to corporate America's profit-based ideals.

Since its inception, the Dove Campaign for Real Beauty has sought to reverse the damaging toll these unrealistic expectations have taken on women. "Imagine a world where beauty is a source of confidence, not anxiety," its motto states. Sounds pretty good. But the reason for its inception is sad. The campaign was the result of a global study conducted in 2004 that showed that only 2 percent of the world's women classified themselves as beautiful. In 2007, another global study, Beauty Comes of Age, revealed that 91 percent of women aged fifty to sixty-four believe it's time for society to change its views about women and aging. Four years later, Dove released the findings of its largest global study to date about women's relationship with beauty—*The Real Truth about Beauty: Revisited*. Results from the study showed that just 4 percent of women around the world consider themselves beautiful, and that anxiety about looks begins in childhood. "In a study of over 1,200 ten to 17-year-olds, a majority of girls, 72 percent, said they felt tremendous pressure to be beautiful," says Dove's website. "The study also found that only 11 percent of girls around the world feel comfortable using the word 'beautiful' to describe their looks, showing that there is a universal increase in beauty pressure and a decrease in girls' confidence as they grow older."[1]

BECOMING REAL

Recovery, or healing, is about daring to become real. Becoming real is about letting go and embracing the plan that was designed for you. It means being able to look in the mirror and like what you see, focusing on those features you admire about yourself, and leaving the rest aside. Your hair may not shine like it used to, but look at your smile! Your wrinkles have deepened, but you've had a lot to laugh about. Your breasts may sag, but they've nourished your babies and a pretty bra is just the trick to make you feel *hot* again. And more than that, becoming real means looking at all the things in your life that enrich you and your family.

Michelle, a former anorexic and a forty-four-year-old mother of three, says, "Becoming real was about . . . [realizing] all of the connections I have in my relationships. My focus on food and weight separated me from those connections, and the people I love, and from myself."

This relationship between love and worth has never been more beautifully illustrated than in the classic children's book *The Velveteen Rabbit*, by Margery Williams:

"What is real?" the Rabbit asked the Skin Horse.

"It doesn't happen all at once," said the Skin Horse. "You become. It takes a long time. That's why it doesn't often happen to people who break easily, or have sharp edges or who have to be carefully kept. Generally, by the time you are Real, most of your hair has been loved off, and your eyes drop out and you get loose in the joints and very shabby. But these things don't matter at all, because once you are Real, you can't be ugly, except to people who don't understand.'"[2]

It's not about one mom standing in front of the mirror. It's about thousands of moms. As women, we are all connected. Your life matters. Your value is worth more than you can imagine. And the lives you're touching are more than you'll ever know.

MORE THAN A SWIMSUIT

When you look in the mirror, do you see wide-set eyes, thin lips, and callused hands? Or do you see irises big enough to absorb God and truth and purity? A mouth that has kissed the same man for years, and hands that have soothed the fevered brows of children grown inside your womb? When you look at your stomach, do you see scars, stretch marks, and excess flab, or the beautiful flesh that surrounded, and opened up for, your babies? Do you see a body that split wide in a gorgeously selfless manner so that others could enter the world? We need to treat ourselves with reverence, for the incredible acts of service our bodies do each day. For the way they allow us to walk, talk, eat, breathe, laugh, run, and hold up our necks. For the simple sensations we so easily take for granted.

"My boys officially smell of summer," Lisa-Jo Baker writes. "And to me, summer smells like sunscreen. The ritual has begun—the spraying and lathering and rubbing into scalps of sweet smelling SPF 50 on blond hair and pale white bodies. . . . They love it. They stand—arms akimbo—and rotate slowly as I mist them. Teeny tiny waists astride gulping swimsuits that all but swallow their cute little patoots; hide their calves and brush just short of their ankles.

". . . We wade into the water together. Their tiny selves next to my not-so-tiny-self. And it makes me proud. Because this body of mine that can't ever seem to find a flattering suit, this body birthed those two boys. This body has seen life that the adorable taut, toned and tiny lifeguard girls on duty couldn't possibly dream of yet.

"This body has housed three miracles and it turns out that miracles need room to grow. This beautiful, amazing body has stretched to accommodate three sets of feet, three heads, three hearts, three sets of flexing limbs. This body is round where some say it should be flat; soft where some say it should be hard; and full where many others are running on empty.

"This body knows what it is. And it is much, much more than a swimsuit."[3]

So let's take it back. Let's take it all back. Our butts, our boobs, our bodies. They belong to us anyway, don't they, girls? It's feminism of the finest kind. A kind that stands up for women, everywhere, of all sizes, shapes, and colors. A kind that sees wrinkles as indicators of a richly lived life; calluses, as places where love has left her signature; lips, as vehicles of kindness; eyes, as windows to the soul; and hands, as instruments of compassion. Our appearance is what we make of it. It belongs to no one but us. So start to look at yourself in a backward kind of way, a holistic kind of way, a loving kind of way. "Now we see things imperfectly, like puzzling reflections in a mirror, but then we will see everything with perfect clarity," writes Paul in 1 Corinthians 13:12. "All that I know now is partial and incomplete, but then I will know everything completely, just as God now knows me completely."

A PERFECT KIND OF LOVE

Sherry sounded just like all the other girls who had contacted Emily through her eating disorders blog, *Chasing Silhouettes*. Sherry wanted to get better, she said, she really did—but she hated herself. And deep down, Emily knew Sherry didn't want to recover, because true healing requires a person deciding that he or she is worth getting better for.

Sherry had been starving herself for years. It started, she said, with peers making fun of her. And so, her self-hatred began, in a form of mutilation that would cut her skin with the edge of a knife if she ate too much. Over time, the pangs of hunger became sharper than the blade. It became a thrilling mission statement, a goal that infused her life with meaning. If Sherry wasn't skinny, she wouldn't matter, or so "the voice" told her.

And she couldn't wait to get to size 1. "But what's after that?" Emily challenged her. "Size 0? And then you die. Do you want to die, Sherry?"

Because when it comes down to it, that's the question: *Do we want to live or die?* Do we believe we are worth the oxygen, the food, the bed, the clothes, the earth's resources required for us to occupy space on this planet? More than food, we hunger for love. And the only love that will ever satisfy is one no human can provide.

"We have an enemy," says youth worker and mother of two Katherine Nanninga. "It is that enemy who steals the joy out of perfect days, who convinces us to hate ourselves . . . our enemy hates us and hates what we can do when we oppose him. I believe he hates families, too, and will do anything to destroy the love and joy that can be experienced within them. He uses our physical, mental and spiritual weaknesses (and even our strengths) against us to destroy the kingdom of God.

And I believe that the first thing he does is to point our anger at God rather than at him, the real source of our pain.

"When we remember who our enemy is and begin our battle against him God helps us to overcome each battle. The big ones and the little ones. I think that each of us fights different little battles but in the big picture, they are all part of the big battle. The joy comes in winning the little battles.

"When we choose to love our children rather than yell (at them), we win, God wins! When we choose to eat well to take care of ourselves and our families we win, God wins! When we choose to rest in God's strength and accept his story for our lives rather than being angry or bitter we win, God wins and our enemy is defeated! So I encourage you to stand up, and let's defeat him! One day our Lord will destroy him and all of our sadness forever. Until then, we are at battle."[4]

GETTING NAKED

Author, pastor, and theologian John Piper said, "The quickest way to the heart is through a wound." This is something that Jillian, a mother to seven children, has been learning over the course of her life. Jillian is a self-proclaimed overachiever. "When it came to dropping the freshman fifteen in college," she says, "I just kept going. It felt like achievement. It felt like discipline. It was so rewarding." But it was also the reason her marriage almost ended in its first year. With a husband who was addicted to Internet porn, Jillian felt in constant competition with the airbrush. "I didn't want to be abandoned, like I had been when I got pregnant at sixteen," she says, "so I had to look better than what was on the screen." Meanwhile, they both worked with youth, and Jillian would compare herself to thirteen- and fourteen-year-old girls. Her eating and exercise regime was strict. "Actually, strict would be a good word for a lot of my life at that point."

But she binged when she was angry. Being in ministry while holding down full-time jobs and attending school, Jillian and her husband battled a lot of stress—and a lot of pressure to hold it together. "I was as strict with him and my expectations of him as I was on myself (don't we all do that projecting thing?). Add that in with ED and sexual addiction and you've got devastation waiting to happen."

But then, she says, God happened. "It took me puking up a delicious Sunday dinner at the home of one of our youth group kids, and then having the toilet stop up and overflow for me to get caught." She was forced to see, for the first time, the ugliness of it all. Meanwhile, Jillian's husband got scared and started trying to control his wife's eating. That, she says, didn't go over well. But it was also the straw that broke the camel's back. They knew they needed help, and they began going to counseling. And they started to learn.

"I have had seven pregnancies in a row, now," says Jillian, "and feel like I am more challenged with my body image than ever. But, oddly, I also feel more grounded in who I am than ever. Like I'm finally getting comfortable in my own skin. Saggy though it is. Maybe some of that overachieving strictness is beginning to be replaced by grace. For myself and for others. Grace is so enlarging, so different from the shriveling, strangling, narrowness of living under laws."

Jillian has been amazed by the way God is redeeming, not only her relationship with herself, but with her husband. "To all husbands, I think, the most beautiful wife is a naked wife," she says. "Not a thin wife. Not a chiseled wife. Not an airbrush. But one who lets him love her . . . sag, stretch marks, and all. And is confident that she will be loved, just as she is. It has revolutionized our intimacy. . . . And is still rocking my understanding of how God wants to love me."

EMILY'S STORY

In spite of knowing God loves me, I wonder. I wake up desiring to do something meaningful, something brilliant and good, and I go to bed wondering if I'll ever live up to my own expectations. And then I say my prayers, whispering belief in the only One who will ever be good enough. *The One whose sole desire for me, every day, is to know how loved I am.*

I am addicted to performing, to proving my worth, and my husband is content just breathing. He reminds me of my son this way, in love with the notion of living and doing it fully: by stretching out on a lawn chair and reading while I run around trying to prove to the world that I matter.

"What is wrong?" he asks when he sees me crying into my cereal. I don't know how to tell him: I'm tired. I may not starve myself anymore, but my anorexic tendencies still show themselves through my need to control. My need to be something more than I am. I want desperately to lie on the lawn chair and read. To hold my babies and breathe in their smell before they grow up. Instead, I do the laundry, work on freelance assignments, and weep.

I am beginning to think maybe it all boils down to this: *life is not about us.* It is not about food. It is about a baby born to save us from all of the sorrow that makes us want to lose ourselves in food. It is about the God-turned-human who delivers us from all of the madness of a world gone wrong. I listen to my husband, a man for whom food has never been anything but a tool for celebration, talk about how much he loves to eat, and I long for his eyes. Eyes that see food as a gift, and our bodies as worthy of that gift. If Trent wants to eat, he eats. He listens to his stomach, and it tells him what it wants—protein, carbs, fruit, and when he's full, he's full. And then he turns and leaves his plate where it belongs—in the sink—and he enjoys the rest of his day without thinking about food once until the next time he's hungry. We need to remember that we were born for more than this world, to see food as just this: a gift. Our bodies as tents of skin, which house the soul.

As psychiatrist and author Elisabeth Kübler-Ross said, "People are like stained-glass windows. They sparkle and shine when the sun is out, but when the darkness sets in, their true beauty is revealed only if there is a light from within."[5]

And so, dear friends, ignite that inner light. And then, just let it shine.

REFLECTION

- Would you say you love yourself? Do you love your whole self, or parts? If so, which parts?
- When you look at yourself in the mirror, do you think kindly about what you see? Or do you tear yourself down?
- How do you qualify your value? What, in your opinion, determines beauty? Which of your attributes would you say are beautiful, and why?

- Do you allow society to determine your opinion of yourself? If so, how and why? Do you long to be set free from society's expectations? Why or why not?
- When you speak love into your children's lives, do you speak the kind that lasts? Or do you subconsciously impose society's expectations on them as well?

TOOLS

- Make a list of what you believe are your best attributes. Then make a list of the other qualities, and compare: which are true by society's standards, and which can be redeemed through a different pair of eyes?
- True identity doesn't just happen. As the Skin Horse said, "You become." It's an evolving process. It begins with the desire to be more than your body, clothes, hair, and weight, even more than your role as a mother. Because you are a woman first. True identity comes about from a place of willingness and introspection. Take time to examine yourself. Spend time alone. Reflect on what you like about yourself and identify your strengths and weaknesses. Know your values and how they line up with your behaviors. Strong principles shape our motivation, decisions, and ultimately, who we are.
- Try new things and activities that bring you joy. It is vital to your sense of well-being and to your growth as a person. You will make mistakes and you will experience loss. But don't be afraid. It is through our mistakes and errors that real growth occurs.
- Every morning, look in the mirror and make a positive affirmation. Make it about more than your physical appearance. Select clothes that reflect your style and taste. Confidence will prevent you from losing sight of who you are.

ACKNOWLEDGMENTS

To our families, who gave up their mommies and wives so we could write about how to be just that—it is your love that makes us live. Thank you.

To our agent, Linda Konner, who believed in the project from day one; to our editor, Suzanne I. Staszak-Silva, who spent hours counseling, guiding, critiquing, and applauding us onward; to our proofreaders, Nicole Myer Unice, MA, LPC, Leanne Spencer, MA, Med, LPC, Lisa-Jo Baker, Amanda Batty, and Helen Burns; and to FINDINGbalance nutrition editor Ann Capper, RD, CDN, who helped us find light and vision—thank you.

To Emme, who humbly cheered us on and breathed life into the manuscript through her foreword, and to all who shared their stories within these pages, who bravely bared their hearts and wounds, thank you.

To our mothers and fathers and sisters and brothers, for loving us in spite of us, and to our friends who believe in us—thank you.

And above all, to the Great I Am, who creates us and saves us from ourselves and makes us whole again. We are dust without you.

Thank you.

APPENDIX

BOOKS

Beating Ana: How to Outsmart Your Eating Disorder and Take Your Life Back, by Shannon Cutts. Health Communications, 2009.

The Body Image Workbook: An Eight-Step Program for Learning to Like Your Looks, 2nd edition, by Thomas F. Cash. New Harbinger Publications, 2008.

The Body Myth: Adult Women and the Pressure to Be Perfect, by Margo Maine. John Wiley & Sons, 2005.

Body Wars: Making Peace with Women's Bodies, by Margo Maine. Gurze Books, 2000.

Breaking Free from Anorexia and Bulimia, by Dr. Linda Mintle. Strang Communications, 2002.

Chasing Silhouettes: How to Help a Loved One Battling and Eating Disorder, by Emily Wierenga. Ampelon Publishing, 2012.

Eating Disorders: A Guide to Medical Care and Complications, by Philip Mehler and Arnold Andersen. Johns Hopkins University Press, 2000.

Handbook of Eating Disorders, 2nd ed., by J. Treasure, U. Schmidt, and E. van Furth (eds). John Wiley & Sons, 2003.

Hollow: An Unpolished Tale, by Jena Morrow. Moody Publishers, 2010.

Hope, Help and Healing for Eating Disorders: A Whole-Person Approach to Treatment of Anorexia, Bulimia and Disordered Eating, by Gregory Jantz, PhD, and Ann McMurray. Waterbrook-Multnomah, 2010.

Life Inside the "Thin" Cage: A Personal Look into the Hidden World of the Chronic Dieter, by Constance Rhodes. Shaw Books, 2003.

Life Without ED: How One Woman Declared Independence from Her Eating Disorder and How You Can Too, by Jenni Schaefer. McGraw-Hill, 2003.
Loving Your Body, by Dr. Deborah Newman. Tyndale, 2002.
Mom, I Feel Fat: Becoming Your Daughter's Ally in Developing a Healthy Body Image, by Sharon A. Hersh. Random House, 2001.
Reviving Ophelia: Saving the Selves of Adolescent Girls, by Mary Pipher. Riverhead Trade, 2005.
Skinny: She Was Starving to Fit In (A Novel), by Laura L. Smith. NAV Press, 2008.
Thin Enough: My Spiritual Journey through the Living Death of an Eating Disorder, by Sheryle Cruse. New Hope Publishers, 2005.
Unsqueezed: Springing Free from Skinny Jeans, Nose Jobs, Highlights and Stilettos, by Margot Starbuck. Inter-Varsity Press, 2010.
Wanting to Be Her: Body Image Secrets Victoria Won't Tell You, by Michelle Graham. Inter-Varsity Press, 2005.
Weightless: Flying Free, Soaring above Food Issues Workbook, by Joni Jones. CarePoint Ministries, 2006.
Weightless: Making Peace with Your Body, by Kate Wicker. Servant Books, 2011.
When Your Child Has an Eating Disorder: A Step-by-Step Workbook for Parents and Other Caregivers, by Abigail Natenshon. John Wiley & Sons, 1999.

WEBSITES

- **Body Image: Loving Your Body Before, During, and After Your Pregnancy**: http://www.americanpregnancy.org/pregnancyhealth/bodyimage.html
  This site discusses the importance of being comfortable with your body before pregnancy. It also explains what you can do to continue to love your body through all the major changes of pregnancy and the postpartum period.
- **Eating Disorder Hope**: http://www.eatingdisorder.com
  Offers information, eating disorder treatment options, recovery tools, and resources for those suffering from eating disorders, as well as for their treatment providers, and loved ones.
- **Eating Disorders during Pregnancy**: http://www.americanpregnancy.org/pregnancyhealth/eatingdisorders.html
  This site explains how eating disorders affect fertility and pregnancy. It also provides information on what you can do to ensure your and your baby's health before, during, and after pregnancy.

- **Eating during Pregnancy**: http://kidshealth.org/parent/nutrition_center/dietary_needs/eating_pregnancy.html
  This site explains the importance of eating well during pregnancy. It includes information about nutrients your body needs, food cravings, and foods and beverages that should be avoided during pregnancy.
- **Eating for Life Alliance:** http://www.eatingforlife.org
  Dedicated to making user-friendly information, resources, protocols, and the wisdom of the nation's experts available to everyone. College is not only a time when eating disorders often develop, but an excellent time to address and heal from them.
- **The Feeding Doctor:** http://www.thefeedingdoctor.com
  Katja Rowell, MD, the Feeding Doctor, who trained under El-lyn Satter, MS, RD, LCSW, BCD, teaches mothers how to feed their families.
- **FINDINGbalance:** http://www.findingbalance.com
  The world's largest media-based resource for people seeking balance with food and body image.
- **Gurze Books**: http://www.bulimia.com
  A bookstore and publisher of information about eating disorders.
- **Healthy Pregnancy**: http://www.womenshealth.gov/pregnancy
  Womenshealth.gov has created this site for expectant mothers. It provides information on fertility and birth control, each trimester of pregnancy, preparing for a new baby, childbirth, postpartum care, and financial help.
- **Maternal and Child Health Bureau, HRSA, HHS**: http://www.mchb.hrsa.gov
  This site provides leadership, in partnership with key stakeholders, and improves the physical and mental health, safety, and well-being of the maternal and child health (MCH) population that includes all the nation's women, infants, children, adolescents, and their families.
- **MentorCONNECT**: http://www.mentorconnect-ed.org
  The first global eating disorders mentoring community and a registered 501(c)3 nonprofit organization.
- **Stretch Marks**: http://www.mayoclinic.com/health/stretch-marks/DS01081

This site gives information about stretch marks, which are common in pregnancy or weight gain. Information includes causes, treatment, and lifestyle remedies for stretch marks.

ORGANIZATIONS

- **Academy for Eating Disorders**: http://www.aedweb.org
  A global professional association committed to leadership in eating disorders research, education, treatment, and prevention.
- **Alliance for Eating Disorders Awareness:** http://www.eating disorderinfo.org, 561-841-0900
- **American Pregnancy Association**: http://www.americanpreg nancy.org
  A national health organization committed to promoting reproductive and pregnancy wellness through education, research, advocacy, and community awareness.
- **Andrea's Voice:** http://andreasvoice.org
- **Binge Eating Disorder Association (BEDA):** http://www .bedaonline.com
- **Compulsive Eaters Anonymous—12-Step Recovery Program:** 310-942-8161
- **The Dressing Room Project:** http://www.thedressingroom project.org, 828-318-4438
- **Eating Disorder Referral and Information Center:** http://www.edreferral.com, 858-481-1515
- **Eating Disorders Action Group:** http://www.e-d-a-g.com, 902-443-9944
- **Eating Disorders Anonymous:** http://www.eatingdisorders anonymous.org
- **Eating Disorders Association of Canada:** http://www.edac-atac .ca
- **Eating Disorders Coalition:** http://www.eatingdisorders coalition.org, 202-543-3842
- **The Elisa Project:** http://www.theelisaproject.org, 214-369-5222

- **Food Addicts Anonymous:** http://www.foodaddictsanonymous .org, 561-967-3871
- **Harvard Eating Disorders Center:** http://www.hedc.org, 888-236-1188
- **Healing Connections, Inc.:** http://www.healingconnections.org, 212-585-3450
- **HUGS International Inc.:** http://www.hugs.com
- **International Association of Eating Disorders Professionals:** http://www.iaedp.com
  A nonprofit providing education and certification, while promoting effective treatment.
- **Jessie's Wish:** http://www.jessieswish.org, 804-378-3032
- **Massachusetts Eating Disorders Association, Inc.:** http://www.medainc.org, 617-558-1881
- **Multi-Service Eating Disorder Association:** http://www .medainc.org
  A nonprofit organization dedicated to the prevention and treatment of eating disorders and disordered eating.
- **National Association to Advance Fat Acceptance, Inc. (NAAFA):** 800-442-1214
- **National Association of Anorexia Nervosa and Associated Disorders, Inc. (ANAD):** http://www.anad.org
  A nonprofit dedicated to the prevention and alleviation of eating disorders since 1976.
- **National Association for Males with Eating Disorders, Inc.:** http://www.namedinc.org, 877-780-0080
- **National Center for Overcoming Overeating:** http://www .overcomingovereating.com, 212-875-0442
- **National Eating Disorders Association (NEDA):** http://www .nationaleatingdisorders.org, 800-931-2237
- **National Eating Disorders Screening Program:** http://www .nmisp.org/eat.htm
- **Overeaters Anonymous:** http://www.overeatersanonymous.org, 505-891-2664

- **Promoting Legislation & Education About Self-Esteem, Inc. (PLEASE):** 860-521-2515
- **Sheena's Place:** http://www.sheenasplace.org
- **WINS—We Insist on Natural Shapes:** http://www.winsnews .org, 800-600-WINS

INTERNATIONAL ORGANIZATIONS

- **British Columbia Eating Disorders Association (Canada):** 250-383-2755
- **Center for the Study of Anorexia and Bulimia (New York):** 212-595-3449
- **Eating Disorders Association (Ireland):** 080-232-234914
- **Eating Disorders Association (UK):** http://www.edauk.com, 01603 621 414
- **Eating Disorders Association (Western Australia):** 9221 0488
- **The National Eating Disorder Information Centre (Canada):** http://www.nedic.ca
- **Somerset & Wessex Eating Disorders Association (UK):** http://www.swedauk.org, 01458 448600

INSTITUTIONS

- **The Center:** http://www.aplaceofhope.com
- **Brookhaven Hospital:** http://www.brookhavenhospital.com
- **Eating Recovery Center:** http://www.eatingrecoverycenter.com
- **Mercy Ministries Canada:** http://www.mercyministries.ca
- **Mercy Ministries USA:** http://www.mercyministries.org
- **Park Nicollet:** http://www.parknicollet.com/medical-services/ eating-disorders
- **Pine Grove:** http://www.pinegrovetreatment.com/womens -center.html
- **The Ranch:** http://www.recoveryranch.com
- **Remuda Ranch:** http://www.remudaranch.com
- **Rock Recovery:** http://www.rockrecoveryed.org
- **Rosewood Centers for Eating Disorders:** http://www.rose woodranch.com

- **Selah House:** http://www.selahhouse.net, 888-641-0022
- **Timberline Knolls:** http://www.timberlineknolls.com
- **Alexian Brothers Behavioral Health Hospital:** Hoffman Estates, IL
- **Avalon Hills:** Utah
- **Casa Palmera:** Del Mar, CA
- **California Baptist University:** Riverside, CA
- **Cedar Springs Austin:** Austin, TX
- **Center for Change:** Orem, UT
- **Center for Discovery/Oceanaire:** Downey, CA
- **Delray Center for Healing:** Delray Beach, FL
- **Eating Disorder Center of Denver:** Denver, CO
- **Eating Recovery Center:** Denver, CO
- **Fairwinds Treatment Center:** Clearwater, FL
- **Focus Center for Eating Disorders:** Chattanooga, TN
- **Insight Psychological Centers, LLC:** Chicago, IL
- **Loma Linda Behavioral Medicine Center:** Loma Linda, CA
- **McCallum Place:** St. Louis, MO
- **New Dawn Eating Disorder Recovery Centers:** Sausalito, CA
- **Oliver-Pyatt Centers:** South Miami
- **Puente de Vida:** California
- **Rader Programs:** California and Oklahoma
- **Ranch 2300:** Lubbock, TX
- **Reasons Eating Disorder Center @ BHC Alhambra Hospital:** Rosemead, CA
- **Rogers Memorial Hospital:** Oconomowoc, WI
- **SeaSide Palm Beach:** West Palm Beach, FL
- **Renfrew Centers:** Pennsylvania and Florida
- **Valenta Eating Disorder Clinic:** Rancho Cucamonga, CA

COUNSELING SERVICES

- **American Association of Christian Counselors:** http://www.aacc.net
- **American Psychological Association:** http://www.apa.org

- **Canadian Counselling and Psychotherapy Association:** http://www.ccacc.ca
- **Canadian Professional Counsellors Association:** http://www.cpca-rpc.ca
- **Professional Association of Canadian Christian Counsellors:** http://www.paccc.ca

NOTES

INTRODUCTION

1. Mothers by the Numbers, http://www.infoplease.com/spot/momcensus1.html.

2. Science Daily, "Three Out of Four American Women Have Disordered Eating, Survey Suggests," April 23, 2008, http://www.sciencedaily.com/releases/2008/04/080422202514.htm.

CHAPTER 1: OUR BODIES, OURSELVES

1. Mary Pipher, *Hunger Pains: The Modern Woman's Tragic Quest for Thinness* (New York: Ballantine Books, 1995), 4.

2. Mary Pipher, *The Shelter of Each Other: Rebuilding Our Families* (New York: Ballantine Books, 1997), 117.

3. Goodreads, "Quotes about Womanhood," http://www.goodreads.com/quotes/tag/womanhood.

4. Goodreads, "Quotes about Womanhood."

5. Anne Lamott, *Plan B: Further Thoughts on Faith* (New York: Riverhead Books, 2005), 171–72.

6. Brandee Shafer, "My Relationship with Food," *Smooth Stones*, March 21, 2012, http://brandeeshafer.blogspot.ca/2012/03/my-relationship-with-food-pt-1.html#disqus_thread.

7. Lamott, *Plan B*, 3–6.

8. PR Newswire, "Leading Eating Disorders Treatment Center, Remuda Ranch, Celebrates International No Diet Day," http://www.prnewswire.com/news-releases/leading-eating-disorders-treatment-center-remuda-ranch-cele brates-international-no-diet-day-120778459.html.

CHAPTER 2: A BRUISED BEGINNING

1. Mary Pipher, *Reviving Ophelia: Saving the Selves of Adolescent Girls* (New York: Riverhead Trade, 2005), 39.

2. Pipher, *Reviving Ophelia*, 21.

3. Anne Lamott, *Grace (Eventually): Thoughts on Faith* (New York: Riverhead, 2007), 74.

4. Mayo Clinic, "Definition," http://www.mayoclinic.com/health/eating-disorders/DS00294.

5. Something Fishy, "Genetics and Biology," http://www.something-fishy.org/isf/genetics.php.

6. BBC News Online Network, "Genetic Clues to Eating Disorders," http://news.bbc.co.uk/2/hi/health/259226.stm.

7. BBC News Online Network, "Brain Chemicals May Cause Bulimia," http://news.bbc.co.uk/2/hi/health/192727.stm.

8. Jenny Deam, "The Scary Rise in Adult Eating Disorders," *Women's Health*, April 2012, http://www.womenshealthmag.com/health/adult-eating-disorders#ixzz1pmqV6d9T.

9. Jenny Deam, "New Eating Disorders," *Women's Health*, April 2012, http://www.womenshealthmag.com/health/new-eating-disorders.

10. Something Fishy, "Eating Disorders Not Otherwise Specified," http://www.something-fishy.org/whatarethey/ednos.php.

CHAPTER 3: FROM BRUISED TO BROKEN

1. Madeleine L'Engle, *Glimpses of Grace: Daily Thoughts and Reflections* (New York: HarperCollins, 1996), 15.

2. Goodreads, "The Shack Quotes," http://www.goodreads.com/work/quotes/2666268-the-shack.

3. "Anne Lamott on Body Image," http://www.beliefnet.com/Video/Beliefnet-Interviews/Anne-Lamott/Anne-Lamott-On-Body-Image.aspx.

4. Anne Lamott, *Traveling Mercies: Some Thoughts on Faith* (New York: Anchor, 2000), 103.

CHAPTER 4: BEFORE AND AFTER

1. Anne Lamott, *Operating Instructions: A Journal of My Son's First Year* (New York: Anchor, 2005), 59.
2. Brandee Shafer, *Smooth Stones*, http://brandeeshafer.blogspot.ca/.
3. C. Berg, L. Togersen, A. Von Holle, R. M. Hamer, C. M. Bulik, and T. Reichborn-Kjennerud, "Factors Associated with Binge Eating Disorder in Pregnancy," *International Journal of Eating Disorders* 44 (March 2011): 124–33.
4. *Dimensions*, "Fired Pregnant Actress Awarded Damages in L.A.," http://www.dimensionsmagazine.com/news/melrose_2.html.
5. Mayo Clinic, "Pregnancy Weight Gain: What's Healthy?" http://www.mayoclinic.com/health/pregnancy-weight-gain/PR00111/NSECTION-GROUP=2.
6. American Pregnancy Association, "Weight Gain with Multiples," http://www.americanpregnancy.org/multiples/weightgain.html.
7. American Pregnancy Association, "About Pregnancy Weight Gain," http://www.americanpregnancy.org/pregnancyhealth/aboutpregweightgain.html.
8. Think Exist, "Elizabeth Stone," http://thinkexist.com/quotes/elizabeth_stone.
9. Lisa-Jo Baker, "It's True What They Say about Childbirth and Then Some," *The Gypsy Mama*, March 29, 2011, http://thegypsymama.com/2011/03/its-true-what-they-say-about-childbirth-and-then-some.
10. National Eating Disorders Association, http://www.nationaleatingdisorders.org; Eating Disorder Referral and Information Center, http://www.edreferral.com.

CHAPTER 5: CHANGE, ACCEPTANCE, AND MORE CHANGE

1. Quote Garden, http://www.quotegarden.com/pregnancy.html.
2. Quote Garden, http://www.quotegarden.com/pregnancy.html.
3. Janae Maslowski, "Birth," *A Woman's Journey*, April 22, 2012, http://janaecharlotte.wordpress.com/2012/04/22/birth.
4. *Scientific American*, "Postpartum Depression Epidemic Affects More Than Just Mom," February 2008, http://www.scientificamerican.com/article.cfm?id=misery-in-motherhood.
5. Brooke Shields, *Down Came the Rain: My Journey through Post-Partum Depression* (New York: Hyperion, 2005).

6. JoAnn Hallum, "When It Rains, and You Cry, and the Clothes Don't Wash Themselves," *Ostriches Look Funny*, April 18, 2012, http://ostricheslook funny.blogspot.ca/2012/04/when-you-cry-and-it-rains-and-clothes.html.

7. Quote Garden, http://www.quotegarden.com/mom-day.html.

CHAPTER 6: THE SLEEPLESS WIFE

1. Quote World, http://www.quoteworld.org/quotes/3293.

2. Emerson Eggerichs, *Love and Respect: The Love She Most Desires; The Respect He Desperately Needs* (Nashville: Thomas Nelson, 2004), 37–38.

3. Think Exist, http://thinkexist.com/quotation/a_successful_marriage_re quires_falling_in_love/157722.html.

CHAPTER 7: BEYOND BREAST MILK (OR FORMULA)

1. Lisa-Jo Baker, "Five Minute Friday—Beauty," *The Gypsy Mama*, August 12, 2011, http://thegypsymama.com/2011/08/five-minute-friday-beauty.

2. Mary Pipher, *Hunger Pains: The Modern Woman's Tragic Quest for Thinness* (New York: Ballantine Books, 1995), 5.

3. Evelyn Tribole, MS, RD, and Elyse Resch, MS, RD, FADA, "10 Principles," http://www.intuitiveeating.org/content/10-principles.

4. Pipher, *Hunger Pains*, 113.

5. Madeleine L'Engle, *Glimpses of Grace: Daily Thoughts and Reflections* (New York: HarperCollins, 1996), 33.

6. Academy of Nutrition and Dietetics, "Eat Right," http://www.eatright.org.

7. Ellyn Satter, RD, *Child of Mine: Feeding with Love and Good Sense* (Boulder, CO: Bull Publishing, 2000), 3.

8. Sandi Richard, "Cooking for the Rushed," http://www.cookingforth erushed.com/new.

CHAPTER 8: FOOD FROM HEAVEN

1. Ann Voskamp, *One Thousand Gifts* (Grand Rapids, MI: Zondervan, 2010), 120.

2. Mental Health Foundation, "The Impact of Spirituality on Mental Health," http://www.rcpsych.ac.uk/pdf/Mental%20Health%20Founda tion%20spirituality%20reportx.pdf.

3. Anne Lamott, *Plan B: Further Thoughts on Faith* (New York: Riverhead Books, 2005), 256.

4. Madeleine L'Engle, *Walking on Water: Reflections on Faith and Art* (New York: Bantam Books, 1980), 230.

5. Think Exist, http://thinkexist.com/quotation/the_mother-child_rela tionship_is_paradoxical_and/147603.html.

6. Sarah Bessey, "In Which You Are Loved and You Are Free," June 6, 2012, http://sarahbessey.com/in-which-you-are-loved-free.

7. Mary Pipher, *Hunger Pains: The Modern Woman's Tragic Quest for Thinness* (New York: Ballantine Books, 1995), 21.

8. Think Exist, http://thinkexist.com/quotation/there_is_a_god_shaped_ vacuum_in_the_heart_of/166425.html.

9. Anne Lamott, *Grace (Eventually): Thoughts on Faith* (New York: Riverhead, 2007), 80.

10. Ann Voskamp, *One Thousand Gifts: The Dare to Live Fully Right Where You Are* (Grand Rapids, MI: Zondervan, 2011), 161.

11. Quote Garden, http://www.quotegarden.com/prayer.html.

12. Think Exist, http://thinkexist.com/quotation/thus-meditating-you-will-no-longer-strive-to/357082.html.

13. Dietrich Bonhoeffer, *Letters and Papers from Prison* (New York: Touchstone, 1997).

CHAPTER 9: LIKE MOTHER, LIKE DAUGHTER

1. Harriet Lerner, PhD, *The Mother Dance: How Children Change Your Life* (New York: Quill, 1998), 185.

2. Lerner, *The Mother Dance*, 190.

3. Lerner, *The Mother Dance*, 192.

4. Anne Lamott, *Operating Instructions: A Journal of My Son's First Year* (New York: Anchor, 2005), 58.

5. Lisa-Jo Baker, "How to Not Splinter Your Daughter's Heart—Epilogue," *The Gypsy Mama*, June 19, 2011, http://thegypsymama.com/2011/06/how-to-not-splinter-your-daughters-heart-epilogue.

6. "Maternal Effects on Daughters' Eating Pathology and Body Image," January 2008, http://www.ncbi.nlm.nih.gov/pubmed/18167323.

7. Lamott, *Operating Instructions*, 158.

CHAPTER 10: BEING THE MIRROR

1. Courtney Walsh, "Training a Daughter Not to Have an Eating Disorder," *Telling Stories,* November 3, 2011, http://courtneywalsh.typepad.com/telling_stories/2011/11/training-a-daughter-not-to-have-an-eating-disorder.html.

2. E. Cooley, T. Toray, M. C. Wang, and N. N. Valdez, "Maternal Effects on Daughters' Eating Pathology and Body Image," *Eating Behaviors* 9 (2008): 52–61.

3. A. Stein, H. Woolley, S. Cooper, J. Winterbottom, C. G. Fairburn, and M. Cortina-Borja, "Eating Habits and Attitudes among 10-Year-Old Children of Mothers with Eating Disorders: Longitudinal Study," *British Journal of Psychiatry* 189 (206): 324–29.

4. Diane Neumark-Sztainer, *I'm Like, So Fat: Helping Your Teen Make Healthy Choices about Eating and Exercise in a Weight-Obsessed World* (New York: Guilford Press, 2005), 46.

5. R. H. Salk and R. Engeln-Maddox, "Frequency, Content, and Impact of Fat Talk among College Women," *Psychology of Women Quarterly* (Evanston, IL: Northwestern University, 2011), 62.

6. Camryn Manheim Quotes, http://www.brainyquote.com/quotes/authors/c/camryn_manheim_2.html.

7. Kathy Kater, *Real Kids Come in All Sizes: 10 Essential Lessons to Build Your Child's Body Esteem* (New York: Broadway, 2004), 86.

8. Darryl Roberts, "The Ugly Truth about America the Beautiful," Huffington Post, August 25, 2008, http://www.huffingtonpost.com/darryl-roberts/the-ugly-truth-about-amer_b_121153.html.

9. Sarah Bessey, "In Which I Promise Not to Call Myself Fat," *The Emerging Mummy,* June 26, 2011, http://tweetmeme.com/story/5560951922/emerging-mummy-in-which-i-promise-not-to-call-myself-fat.

CHAPTER 11: THE ANXIOUS MOTHER

1. Goodreads, http://www.goodreads.com/author/quotes/27399.Debra_Ginsberg.

2. Anxiety and Depression Association of America Screening Tool, "Everyday Anxiety or an Anxiety Disorder?" (2010–2012), http://www.adaa.org/understanding-anxiety.

3. Anxiety and Depression Association of America (2010–2012), http://www.adaa.org/understanding-anxiety.

4. The Free Dictionary, "Anxiety Disorders," http://medical-dictionary .thefreedictionary.com/anxiety+disorders.

5. Anxiety and Depression Association of America (2010–2012), http:// www.adaa.org/understanding-anxiety.

6. Mental Help, "Parents' Anxiety Disorders and Children's Adjustment," http://www.mentalhelp.net/poc/view_doc.php?type=doc&id=13447.

7. *Time*, "Roaring Tigers, Anxious Choppers," January 29, 2011, http:// www.time.com/time/magazine/article/0,9171,2043430,00.html.

8. BDN Maine Health, "To Stressed-Out American Mothers: Try Being French," March 4, 2012, http://bangordailynews.com/2012/03/04/health/to-stressed-out-american-mothers-try-being-french/.

9. N. T. Godart, M. F. Flament, Y. Lecrubier, and P. Jeammet, "Anxiety Disorders in Anorexia Nervosa and Bulimia Nervosa: Co-morbidity and Chronology of Appearance," *International Journal of Eating Disorders* 15 (August 23, 2002): 38–45.

10. W. H. Kaye, C. M. Bulik, L. Thornton, N. Barbarich, and K. Masters, Price Foundation Collaborative Group, "Comorbidity of Anxiety Disorders with Anorexia and Bulimia Nervosa," *American Journal of Psychiatry* 161 (2004): 2215–21.

CHAPTER 12: FRIENDLY COMPETITION

1. Rachel H. Salk and Renee Engeln-Maddox, "If You're Fat, Then I'm Humongous," *Psychology of Women Quarterly* 35, no. 1 (March 2011): 18–28, http://171.67.121.89/content/35/1/18.full.

2. CJ Styles, http://www.cjstyles.com.

3. Harriet Lerner, PhD, *The Mother Dance: How Children Change Your Life* (New York: Quill, 1998), 192.

4. Bruno Monsaingeon, "Picks and Pans Review: Mademoiselle: Conversations with Nadia Boulanger," *People*, September 23, 1985, http://www.people .com/people/archive/article/0,,20091763,00.html.

CHAPTER 13: AS THEY GROW

1. Kathryn Zerbe, MD, *The Body Betrayed: A Deeper Understanding of Women, Eating Disorders and Treatment*, (Carlsbad, CA: Gurze, 1993).

2. Brainy Quote, http://www.brainyquote.com/quotes/authors/v/virginia_satir.html.

3. Quote Garden, http://www.quotegarden.com/teen-drivers.html.

4. Gary Chapman, PhD, and Ross Campbell, MD, *The Five Love Languages of Children* (Chicago: Moody, 2008), 109–11.

5. Chapman and Campbell, *Love Languages*, 115.

6. Lisa-Jo Baker, "Remembering to Like Your Kids and Not Just Love Them," *The Gypsy Mama*, May 5, 2011, http://thegypsymama.com/2011/05/remembering-to-like-your-kids-and-not-just-love-them.

7. Harriet Lerner, PhD, *The Mother Dance: How Children Change Your Life* (New York: Quill, 1998), 192.

8. Goodreads, "Plato Quotes," http://www.goodreads.com/author/quotes/879.Plato.

9. James Dobson, *Bringing Up Boys: Practical Advice and Encouragement for Those Shaping the Next Generation of Men* (Wheaton, IL: Tyndale, 2001), 90.

CHAPTER 14: GETTING HELP

1. Carolyn Costin and Gwen Schubert Grabb, *8 Keys to Recovery from an Eating Disorder: Effective Strategies from Therapeutic Practice and Personal Experience* (New York: W. W. Norton, 2011), 15–16.

2. Costin and Grabb, *8 Keys to Recovery*, 16.

3. Valerie Monroe, "Stop Being So Hard on Yourself," *O, The Oprah Magazine*, June 2008, http://www.oprah.com/spirit/Stop-Being-So-Hard-on-Yourself-Os-Beauty-Revolution_1/2 (accessed March 15, 2012).

4. Lisa Bevere, *You Are Not What You Weigh: End Your War with Food and Discover Your True Value* (Lake Mary, FL: Siloam Press, 2007), 6.

5. American Psychiatric Association, "Practice Guidelines," http://www.psychiatryonline.com/pracGuide/pracGuideTopic_12.aspx.

6. National Eating Disorders Association, *Navigator Handbook* (New York: NEDA, 2009), 7.

7. National Eating Disorders Association, *Navigator Handbook*, 7.

CHAPTER 15: IDENTITY CRISIS

1. Dove, "The Dove Campaign for Real Beauty," http://www.dove.us/Social-Mission/campaign-for-real-beauty.aspx.

2. Margery Williams, *The Velveteen Rabbit* (New York: Smithmark, 1995), 6–7.

3. Lisa-Jo Baker, "You Are More Than Your Swim Suit," *The Gypsy Mama*, May 31, 2011, http://thegypsymama.com/2011/05/you-are-more-than-your-swim-suit.

4. "Imperfect Prose: If God Is So Good and Caring and Loving, Then Why?" http://www.emilywierenga.com/2012/06/if-god-is-so-good-and-caring-and-loving.html.

5. Think Exist, "Elisabeth Kübler-Ross Quotes," http://thinkexist.com/quotation/people_are_like_stained-glass_windows-they/8840.html.

SELECTED
BIBLIOGRAPHY

Bevere, Lisa. *You Are Not What You Weigh: End Your War with Food and Discover Your True Value.* Lake Mary, FL: Siloam Press, 2007.

Chapman, Gary, PhD, and Ross Campbell, MD. *The Five Love Languages of Children.* Chicago: Northfield Publishing, 1997.

Dobson, Dr. James. *Bringing Up Boys: Practical Advice and Encouragement for Those Shaping the Next Generation of Men.* Wheaton, IL: Tyndale, 2001.

Eggerichs, Dr. Emerson. *Love and Respect: The Love She Most Desires; The Respect He Desperately Needs.* Nashville: Thomas Nelson, 2004.

Kater, Kathy. *Real Kids Come in All Sizes: 10 Essential Lessons to Build Your Child's Body Esteem.* New York: Broadway, 2004.

Lamott, Anne. *Plan B: Further Thoughts on Faith.* New York: Riverhead Books, 2005.

———. *Operating Instructions: A Journal of My Son's First Year.* New York: Anchor, 2005.

———. *Traveling Mercies: Some Thoughts on Faith.* New York: Anchor, 2000.

L'Engle, Madeleine. *Glimpses of Grace: Daily Thoughts and Reflections.* New York: HarperCollins, 1996.

———. *Walking on Water: Reflections on Faith and Art.* Colorado Springs: WaterBrook Press, 2001.

Lerner, Harriet, PhD. *The Mother Dance: How Children Change Your Life.* New York: Quill, 1998.

Maine, Margo, PhD. *Father Hunger: Fathers, Daughters and the Pursuit of Thinness.* Carlsbad, CA: Gurze Books, 2004.

National Eating Disorders Association (NEDA). *Navigators Guidebook*. New York: NEDA, 2010.

Neumark-Sztainer, Diane. *I'm Like, So Fat: Helping Your Teen Make Healthy Choices about Eating and Exercise in a Weight-Obsessed World*. New York: Guilford Press, 2005.

Pipher, Mary. *Hunger Pains: The Modern Woman's Tragic Quest for Thinness*. New York: Ballantine Books, 1995.

———. *Reviving Ophelia: Saving the Selves of Adolescent Girls*. New York: Riverhead Trade, 2005.

———. *The Shelter of Each Other: Rebuilding Our Families*. New York: Ballantine Books, 1997.

Satter, Ellyn. *Child of Mine: Feeding with Love and Good Sense*. Boulder, CO: Bull, 2000.

Voskamp, Ann. *One Thousand Gifts: A Dare to Live Fully Right Where You Are*. Grand Rapids, MI: Zondervan, 2011.

Williams, Margery. *The Velveteen Rabbit*. New York: Smithmark, 1995.

INDEX

abandonment, fear of, 192
abuse, 17; bullying, 1; drugs, 95; self, 18; sexual, 18
acceptance: of body image, 173–178; of friendships, 156; of help, 156; parents' of their children, 173–178; of self, 109, 156, 173–178
accountability, in relation to healing, 177
achievement, regarding eating disorders, 192
addiction, sexual, 192
admiration, towards men/husbands, 69
adolescence, 17; versus adulthood, 23
adoption, failed, 45, 147
adulthood, 27, 33
advertising, 127
affection, 141
affirmation, 100; in regards to children, 100, 121; of self, 120, 185; verbal, 130, 165
airbrushing, 127
America the Beautiful, 126–127
American Psychiatric Association (APA), 181

anger, 192
anorexia athletica, 22
anorexia nervosa, 194; in children, 19; as a mental illness, 21, 45; the relapse of, 26, 32
anxiety, xiii; biological basis of, 139; disorder and symptoms of, 137–141; and faith, 92; about feeding children, 77; of motherhood and parenting, 135, 142, 162; in relation to Dove's global studies, 188; in relation to eating disorders, 31, 82, 136, 143; stats, 138; tips for combatting, 137, 145
apology, in relation to children, 115, 161, 167
appearance, 191; according to Mary Pipher and North American culture, 78
appreciation, 69

baby, 55; blues, 53; moon, 55
Baker, Lisa-Jo, 44, 75, 78, 110, 165, 190
balance, finding, 83, 176

beauty, 19, 113, 46, 189; how to inspire, 117, 121; inner, 93, 125, 157, 193; outer, 187, 193; of soul and body, 75, 100

belief: in God and others, 108, 113; in self, 65, 108

Bessey, Sarah, on caring for ourselves as women, 97–98; a letter to her daughters, 128–131

Bevere, Lisa, on the ED identity being a lie, 179

Bible, 91

binge eating disorder, 22

birth, 49

blame, 166, 174

body: appreciation for, 153; overcoming fears of, 114, 120; as a physical container for spiritual souls, 96; post-baby, 64; pre-pregnancy, 38; respect of, 80, 188, 190;

body image: xi, 1, 6, 7, 23, 188; Australian study, 10; and eating disorders, 21; negative, 42; in regards to teenagers, 10; re-shaping, 96; tips for improving, 132–133

body mass index (BMI), 5, 41

Bonhoeffer, Dietrich, 103

breastfeeding, 36; formula, 73; purging via, 76

bulimia nervosa, 21

bullying, 128

Capper, Ann, RD, CDN, 76

celebrity, in relation to pregnancy, 38

change, learning to deal with, 68, 97

Chapman, Gary, and Ross Campbell, 164

Chasing Silhouettes, 191

childbirth, 51

childhood, 113, 167

children, 6, 94; effect of anxiety on, 142; beauty, 110, 121; becoming like, 96; feeding, 77–86; learning from, 97; their love languages, 99, 147, 164–166; and temper tantrums, 147; trusting, 86; turned teenagers, 161, 163, 162, 166–170

choice, overwhelming, 165

chronic dieting, 22

Chua, Amy, 142

co-creators, in relation to women, 95

commitment, demonstrating to children, 123–124

communication, 172; effect of anxiety on, 141; in marriage , 68; with offspring, 136–137; tools for promoting, 131

community, importance of, 61

comparisons, amongst women, 98, 152–154; how society profits from, 188

compassion, inspiring in children, 102

conception, 57

condemnation, towards self and others, 144, 156

confidence, inspiring in children, 193

connection, in relation to family, 189; disconnection, 6, 11; in relation to disordered eating, 122; the lack of when child is born, 50; in soul and body, 6

control, 177; lack of, 50, 135, 169; surrendering, 60

coping, with change, 36

cosmetics industry, lies spread by, 27

Costin, Carolyn, 175

courage, inspiring in children, 121–122

creation, 29, 44

creator, 29, 192

culture, effect on women's identity, 97, 142

daughters, 110; inspiring beauty within,117–118, 136–137; a letter to, 128–131; relationship with fathers, 128; study of mothers and,110

death, spiritual and physical, 95, 108, 137, 191

delegation, within the family, 68

delivery, of a child, 50

Dena's story, 8, 58–60, 85, 112

depression, coping with, 3, 28

diabulimia, 22

dieting, about, 8, 74; effect of, on children, 18, 81, 125; fad, 37; postpartum, 4–5; rejecting the mentality, 79

disordered eating, 7, 9, 11, 18–19, 173; and anxiety, 136–141; versus eating disorders, 22; effect on family, 76,78, 119 , 122, 193; motherhood's effect on, 54; in relation to disordered thinking, 61; triggers of, 28, 157, 161

disordered feeding, 76–77

doctor: communication with, 39, 48; pregnancy visits, 42

Dove Campaign for Real Beauty, 188

drunkorexia, 22

DSM-IV, criteria of, 20–23

eating, 74; versus grazing, 77; intuitive, 78; as a moral issue, 81

eating disorders, xi, xii, 18, 20–23, 118, 125; death from, 9; versus disordered eating, 22; guilt, anxiety over, 31, 77; and infertility, menstrual cycles, 57; and marriage, 193; during pregnancy, 37; recovery from, 43, 173, 176; triggers, 154–155, 157, 162, 170, 174

EDNOS, 22

Eggerichs, Emerson, PhD, 69–70

Emily's story, 24–25, 30–32, 44–46, 56, 65, 82–83, 91, 99–100, 109–112, 146–148, 157, 170, 176, 184, 193

emotional eating, 22; breeding it in children, 76, 180; overcoming, 180

emotions, coping with, 55, 135, 177

Ephron, Nora, on pregnancy, 50

exercise, 8, 19, 21–22, 54; and combatting anxiety, 150; enjoyment, motivation for, 80; moderation in, 10; as a mother, 55

existence, on how it's meaningful, 75

expectations: and God, 193; and motherhood, 166; of self and others, 61, 86

faith, in God, 93–94, 192

family: eating together, 86; finding identity as, 93; involvement with treatment, 182; raising a beauty-full one, 121–124; versus ministry, 100

fathers, in relation to daughters, 128

fat talk, 152–154

fear: of aging, weight-gain, rejection, 112–113, 130; of our children's pain, 171; versus love, 108; how a mother's affects her children, 110, 114, 122; in relation to society, 127; of self, others, 107

feeding, in relation to children, 73–74; according to Ellyn Satter, RD, *The Feeding Doctor*, 86; how-to, 77, 84

feelings, 80, 153–154, 180

feminism, 190

FINDINGbalance, 76

food: challenging the police, 79; in relation to children, 73–74; as a love letter, 82–83, 86; spiritual versus physical, 180

forgiveness, 115, 161, 180

foster care, in relation to Emily's story, 147–148

friendship, 151, 154–155

fullness, satiation, 79

generalized anxiety disorder (GAD), 140

generosity, 103, 155

genes, 7, 174

God: faith in, 93; forgiveness from, 91; humanity's need for, 29, 170, 179; the fulfillment of his love, 33; versus Satan, 192

grace: for each other, 154; for yourself, 157; versus guilt, 174; versus self-judgment, 144, 194;

gratitude: attitude of, 155, 168; importance of practicing daily, 156; inspiring in our children, 103; secret of, 90, 101

guilt, xiii, 55, 141, 166

Hallum, Joann, on motherhood, sadness and faith, 54

happiness, 2, 43, 67

Harriet Lerner, on mothers and daughters, 105–106, 108, 155, 166

healing: from disordered eating, 173, 178; holistic, 175, 189; difficulty of, 174; proactive versus reactive, 176

health: inspiring, 118–121 and love, 30; mental and spiritual, 46, 92; obesity, 11; and pregnancy, 39, 43

history, accepting, 106, 108

hobbies, 67

homeschooling, 100

hope, 170

hormones, and eating disorders, 21

humility, in motherhood, 89, 152; meaning in, 194; in relationships, 156; spiritual healing from, 101–102

hunger, 79, 185

hurting, when your child is, 94

husband, role of, 64–66; involving, 86; making yours matter, 67–68

identity: as defined by disordered eating, 179, 185; impact of negative messages on, 119; nurturing and fostering in selves and children, 124–126; as a pregnant woman, 45; spiritual, 29, 171; value of, xi, 29

imperfection, 108, 195

infertility, 57, 147

institutions, eating disorder, xii, xiii

intuitive eating: during pregnancy, 39, 45; ten steps of, 79–81;

tips for, 132; trusting it in our children, 81

jealousy: effect on families and children of, 151–152; of your children, 162–163; piggybacking on others' identities, 157
journaling, 16

Kater, Kathy, on true identity, 86

labor, 35, 50
Lamaze class, and other ideals of pregnancy, 49
Lamott, Anne, 2, 19, 45, 30, 33, 67, 93, 100, 109
legacy, leaving one for your children, 155–156
L'Engle, Madeleine, 29, 82, 94
lies, 106, 129, 145, 179
life, 96, 191
Loren, Sophia, 58
love, 29, 30, 69, 70, 101, 121, 108, 145, 165, 170; of self, food, children, husband, 83, 95, 148, 155, 158, 163–164
Lush, Jean, 168

Manheim, Camryn, 126
marriage, after childbirth, 63–64; sacrifice and servant-hood required of, 71; self-esteem/EDs and, 28, 31–32, 113;
Maslowski, Janae, 51
maternity, leave, 59
Maudsley Method, Hospital, 21
Mayo Clinic, 20, 39
mealtimes: importance to family, 5, 87; purpose of, connection with,

81; snacking versus, 137; stats, studies regarding, 87
meals: making to-do lists, 86; planning during pregnancy, 47; preparation and disordered feeding, 77
media, 7; effects of, 11, 82, 98, 179; learning to recognize its voice, 107; rejecting its message and teaching our children to as well, 111, 131
medication, side effects of, 138
men, in their role as husbands, 64, 66, 70
mental illness, 18, 21, 137–139, 176
menu, during pregnancy, 41; spiritual, 102
ministry, negative effects of, 25, 100
mirror, reflection, 4, 97, 98, 118
miscarriage, 3, 45; Emily's, 58, 94, 101, 147
mother: Emily's relationship with, 109; in relation to food, body image, 106; guilt, 31; habits to model health and inspire beauty, 118–121; how their eating behaviors affect daughters, 110, 119; a letter from one to her daughters, 128–131; martyr-syndrome, 52; on becoming ours, 100; rejection of by son, 168; role and impact of, 10, 105; separating issues from daughters, 118; study of daughters and, 110
motherhood, uncontrollable aspects of, 19; fears of, 58, 136; the mission of, 54, 65, 90, 96; the sacrifice of, attachment to, 52

NEDA (National Eating Disorder Association), 181–182

negative thoughts, overcoming, 146

neglect, its effect on children, 46

Neumark-Sztainer, Diane, 46

nourishment, spiritual, 93, 141

nutrition, during pregnancy, 35–36, 41; in relation to infants/children, 73

obesity, health problems with, 11; culture's condemnation of, 126

obsessive-compulsive disorder (OCD), 143

overeating, during pregnancy, 39

parenting, xiii, 46; extreme testing of during teenage years, 169; and choosing grace, 91, 144, 167; messiness of, Savior complex, 93; western helicopter type, 143

Pascal, Blaise, 99

past, making peace with, 109; on how it affects our identity, 180

peer pressure, during pregnancy, 42

people-pleasing, in relation to eating disorders, 25

Perfect Mommy Syndrome, 53

personality, prone to anxiety and EDs, 143

perspective, 96, 171, 187, 189

physical touch, 171

Piper, John, 192

Pipher, Mary, on girls growing up, 17; on body image problems, 1, 2; on eating disorders and North American culture, 78; on

encouraging health within our families, 81; tips on body image, 98–99

pleasure, discovering the satisfaction factor, 80

postpartum issues, 37, 52, 53, 59

prayer, 47, 60, 102

pregnancy, effect of EDs on, 31; before and after, 35; comparisons among women, 151; eating during, 37, 41; expected weight gain, 40–41; guidelines for, 47; on how it is creation, 44; on how it can trigger an ED, 37; inspires health, 43; on having multiples, 41

pregorexia, 22

professionals, involved in treatment, 87, 181–182

purpose, beyond appearance, 178

real, on becoming, and how it's the key to recovery and healing, 187–190

recovery, 173–178; Emily's story of, 184–185; issues behind the illness, 185; on how it's a choice, 174; the ten phases of, no quick fixes for, 175; spiritual versus physical, 178

redemption, 107

reflection, and learning to love ours, 67; in our children's lives, 97; traits to focus on, 98

relapse, during pregnancy, 39; chances of, 176; Emily's story of, 184; during marriage, 70

relationship, between food and body, 5; with God, 123; how they are eternal, 151; between mothers and

daughters, 105–106; dependent on repentance and forgiveness, 90–91; between teenagers and parents, 169
respect, towards husband, 69
restrictive eating, 22, 28
Richards, Sandi, 86
Roberts, Darryl, 126–127
romance, 67, 68

sadness, during pregnancy, 43
satisfaction, personal, and how it affects our relationships with others, 152
Satter, Ellyn, RD, 86
scale, doctor's, 9
Schwartz, Allan, LCSW, 141
self-esteem, 7, 35, 119; caring for, 55, 61, 64–65, 66, 118–121, 123, 136–137, 185; distorted perception of, 84, 107, 187; doubt, love of, 1, 2, 11, 40, 28, 36, 83, 177; hatred of, 28, 57; shame of, mistrust of, 74, 152; society's distorted view of, 23, 107
sex, 63–64
sexy, 130
Shafer, Brandee, 3, 36
shame, 113
Shields, Brooke, 53
skinny, 57
society, 4, 23, 38, 39, 61, 187
Something Fishy website, 21
sons, adolescent, 168
spirituality, 26, 60–62, 90–91; according to the Mental Health Foundation, 96, 141; versus physicality, 178; the quiet voice of,

89; in treatment, 182; what it tells us about our worth, 75, 89, 92
starving for love, 25
statistics, diet, 5
Stone, Elizabeth, 42
stress, 28, 74, 138
stretch marks, 23, 63, 111, 190
suffering, when your child is, 94
Surrey, Janet, 122–123
survey, in *Self* magazine, 5
swimsuits, 190

teenagers, 162, 163, 167, 169, 172
therapy, 107, 183
treatment, for EDs, 46, 173–178; advice for finding, 182; questions to consider when choosing, 183–184
triggers, 28, 37, 39, 177
trust, teenagers and, 169
truth, 75, 106, 125
Tylo, Hunter, 38

value, helping our children understand theirs; 129rooted in spirituality, 89, 177
Voskamp, Ann, 90, 101

Wallace, William Ross, 4
Walsh, Courtney, 117
weight, baby, 4–5; postpartum, 6; programs, 8
western worldview, 107; helicopter parenting, 142
wives, role of, 64–66
womanhood, 10; as concealed by cosmetics, 27; effects of pregnancy on, 35

women, their tendency to "break," 66; as heartbeat of the home, 107; taking pride in our stories, 130

worrying, 84

worth, 75, 92, 129

Young, William Paul, 29

Zerbe, Kathryn, PhD, on older women mourning the loss of youth, 163

About the Authors

Dena Cabrera, PsyD, is a licensed clinical psychologist and a certified eating disorder specialist at the Rosewood Centers for Eating Disorders in Wickenburg, Arizona, where she is currently the clinical director of adolescent services. She has personally treated hundreds of women and teens struggling with eating and body image issues. Rosewood Centers for Eating Disorders has served as a distinguished leader in eating disorder treatment for more than a decade. Cabrera is a well-known expert and speaker in the field; she has spoken at more than twenty national conferences and presented more than a hundred workshops on eating disorders and other mental health problems. Cabrera writes articles for magazines, develops news segments for television shows, consults with professionals across the country on eating disorder issues, hosts teleseminars and podcasts, and develops presentations based on cutting-edge research and clinical experience. Cabrera lives in Arizona with her husband and two children.

Emily Wierenga, who battled anorexia both as a child and an adult, was told she would never bear children. Today, Wierenga is a married mother of two boys, as well as a foster mother. She serves as an Official Ambassador for FINDINGbalance and a trained Navigator with the National Eating Disorders Association (NEDA), and has shared her story multiple times on Canada's number-one Christian television talk show, as well as on the nation's most popular spiritual talk-back radio program. In June 2011, she spoke alongside her father at Hungry for

Hope: A Family Affair. She also speaks regularly to women's groups and church groups across the nation. Wierenga is the author of *Save My Children* (Castle Quay Books, 2008) and *Chasing Silhouettes: How to Help a Loved One Battling an Eating Disorder*, with Dr. Gregory Jantz (Ampelon Publishing, 2012). An award-winning freelance journalist, Wierenga is a monthly columnist for the *Christian Courier*, as well as a regular contributor to *A Deeper Story*, *Prodigal Magazine*, *She Loves*, and *The High Calling*. In her free time, she does painting commissions. Wierenga lives in Alberta, Canada, with her husband, Trenton, and their sons. For more information, please visit www.emilywierenga.com.